'The authors of this book are well known ACT therapists, trainers and researchers, in the Dutch community and some beyond. This English edition provides caregivers from other countries a chance to profit from their knowledge and experience. The book shows why clients do what they do, with clear analyses based on ACT and the relational frame theory. Through case descriptions with well-chosen interventions, it becomes clear how ACT can be a fluid process, closely linked to the client's experience. This approach gives ACT therapists the support and freedom they need, to find their own style in working with ACT.'

Jacqueline A-Tjak, *PhD, clinical psychologist and peer-reviewed ACT trainer, author of several books and articles on ACT*

'This book is unique amongst ACT books. Rather than present a set of interventions and metaphors in the form of a protocol, it helps readers relate their ACT practice to underlying processes rooted in Relational Frame Theory. This book will help you ground your clinical practice in basic processes, and increase your clinical mastery and effectiveness.'

Benjamin Schoendorff *is a clinical psychologist and founder of the Contextual Psychology Institute in Montreal. He is peer-reviewed ACT trainer, certified FAP trainer and World Expert in PBBT. He has authored several books for clinicians and the general public.*

'If you're searching for a superb resource to bridge the realms of science and heart in Acceptance and Commitment Therapy (ACT) while enriching your expertise and grasp of this intervention, then ACT with Head and Heart: Working Process-based with Acceptance and Commitment Therapy is the ideal book for you. This book offers an inspirational exploration of ACT intertwined with fundamental behavioral principles. It expertly navigates readers through the practical application of ACT, harnessing the potency of experiential techniques and striving for genuine, transformative change. This book is essential for therapists dedicated to elevating their ACT practice.'

Robyn D. Walser, *PhD, Author of The Heart of ACT, and coauthor of Learning ACT, 2nd Edition and The Mindful Couple, Assistant Professor, University of California, Berkeley.*

W0234989

Practicing Acceptance and Commitment Therapy with Head and Heart

This book will help readers balance the essential scientific concepts underlying Acceptance and Commitment Therapy (ACT) with their clinical practice, reconnecting ACT with its behavioural therapeutic roots and Relational Frame Theory.

Clinicians often struggle to understand the science (the "head") that should underpin their clinical practice/work (the "heart"). Without a core understanding of the scientific concepts underlying ACT, clinicians struggle to understand how to adapt ACT in practice for specific client or group situations and why. In response to that, this book is structured to help readers understand the why of each intervention and how to use that to guide the next move. Through a mix of explanations, personal examples, exercises for the therapist, short cases, and metaphors, the book provides a series of science-driven concepts that teach the reader to use the ACT toolbox with skilful interventions.

This manual is a must-read for any ACT trainee or practitioner, helping them systematically connect techniques with the rationale for their use.

Lieve Bruyninx is the owner of Factor Psy, a mental health care training institute. She is a psychologist and peer-reviewed ACT trainer with 20 years of behaviour therapy expertise.

Yvonne Barnes-Holmes is the Co-Founder of Perspectives Ireland and Co-Developer of Process-Based Behaviour Therapy (PBBT). She has 25 years of experience in behaviour therapy.

Ciara McEnteggart is the Co-Founder of Perspectives Ireland and Co-Developer of Process-Based Behaviour Therapy (PBBT). She has 15 years of experience in behaviour therapy.

Marjolein Vleugel has been working as a Healthcare Psychologist for more than 20 years. She is the founder and head trainer of Expertise Centrum ACT.

Roy Thewissen, PhD, is a clinical psychologist and behavioural therapist. He works as a freelancer and in the pain department at Adelante rehabilitation clinic in the Netherlands.

Practicing Acceptance and Commitment Therapy with Head and Heart

Understanding the Why Behind Each Intervention

Lieve Bruyninx, Yvonne Barnes-Holmes, Ciara McEnteggart, Marjolein Vleugel, and Roy Thewissen

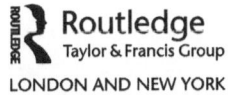

Routledge
Taylor & Francis Group

LONDON AND NEW YORK

Designed cover image: © Getty Images

First English edition published 2025
by Routledge
4 Park Square, Milton Park, Abingdon, Oxon, OX14 4RN

and by Routledge
605 Third Avenue, New York, NY 10158

Routledge is an imprint of the Taylor & Francis Group, an informa business

First Dutch edition published *ACT met hoofd en hart* © 2022 L. Bruyninx, Y. Barnes-Holmes,
C. McEnteggart, R. Thewissen & M. Vleugel p/a Boom Uitgevers Amsterdam

Originally published by Boom uitgevers Amsterdam

British Library Cataloguing-in-Publication Data
A catalogue record for this book is available from the British Library

Library of Congress Cataloging-in-Publication Data
Names: Bruyninx, Lieve, 1974– author. | Barnes-Holmes, Yvonne, author. | McEnteggart, Ciara, 1987–
author. | Vleugel, Marjolein, 1974– author. | Thewissen, Roy, 1977– author. Title: Practicing acceptance
and commitment therapy with head and heart: understanding the why behind each intervention / Lieve
Bruyninx, Yvonne Barnes-Holmes, Ciara McEnteggart, Marjolein Vleugel, Roy Thewissen.
Other titles: ACT met hoofd en hart. English
Description: First English edition. | Abingdon, Oxon ; New York, NY: Routledge, 2025. | First Dutch
edition published as ACT met hoofd en hart. Amsterdam: Boom, 2022. | Includes bibliographical
references and index. | Summary: "This book will help readers balance the essential scientific concepts
underlying Acceptance and Commitment Therapy (ACT) with their clinical practice, reconnecting
ACT with its behavioural therapeutic roots and Relational Frame Theory. Clinicians often struggle to
understand the science (the "head") that should underpin their clinical practice/work (the "heart").
Without a core understanding of the scientific concepts underlying ACT, clinicians struggle to understand
how to adapt ACT in practice for specific client or group situations and why. In response to that, this
book is structured to help readers understand the why of each intervention and how to use that to guide
the next move. Through a mix of explanations, personal examples, exercises for the therapist, short cases,
and metaphors, the book provides a series of science-driven concepts that teach the reader to use the
ACT toolbox with skilful interventions. This manual is a must-read for any ACT trainee or practitioner,
helping them systematically connect techniques with the rationale for their use"— Provided by publisher.
Identifiers: LCCN 2024021335 (print) | LCCN 2024021336 (ebook) | ISBN 9781032699677 (hardback) |
ISBN 9781032672786 (paperback) | ISBN 9781032699691 (ebook)
Subjects: MESH: Acceptance and Commitment Therapy—methods
Classification: LCC RC489.A32 B78 2025 (print) | LCC RC489.A32 (ebook) |
NLM WM 425.5.C6 | DDC 616.89/1425—dc23/eng/20240701
LC record available at https://lccn.loc.gov/2024021335
LC ebook record available at https://lccn.loc.gov/2024021336

ISBN: 9781032699677 (hbk)
ISBN: 9781032672786 (pbk)
ISBN: 9781032699691 (ebk)

DOI: 10.4324/9781032699691

Typeset in Times New Roman
by codeMantra

Contents

About the authors

Lieve Bruyninx

Occupation: Company director of Factor Psy

Lieve Bruyninx is a psychologist and a recognized behavioral therapist with the Flemish Association for Behavioral Therapy. She graduated from the University of Ghent in 1997. She is an experienced therapist who has been working with acceptance and commitment therapy (ACT) since 2006. She is currently integrating relational frame theory (RFT), behavior therapy, and ACT into all aspects of her therapeutic work. As a result, her supervision and training work reflect a strong focus on functional analysis and basic behavioral processes, with the aim of always facilitating transformative individual change and therapeutic skills. She has built up specific expertise in experiential work, the use of metaphors, and creating a safe therapeutic relationship. Lieve is a peer-reviewed ACT trainer and a process-based behavior therapy (PBBT) expert practitioner. She has 20 years of experience in behavior therapy.

Yvonne Barnes-Holmes

Occupation: Company Co-director of Perspectives Ireland

Dr. Yvonne Barnes-Holmes is a chartered behavioral psychologist with the Psychological Society of Ireland. She was a former senior research fellow and associate professor of behavior analysis at Ghent University. She was formerly tenured faculty, including Head of Department, at the Department of Psychology, National University of Ireland, Maynooth. She graduated from the latter in 2001 after completing an experimental Ph.D. She has been involved in attracting 4 million+ euros in funding. She has graduated with 19 doctorates and 7 masters. She has published two books and three edited volumes, 150+ articles and book chapters, and given 500+ talks and workshops, all of which focus on behavioral science, especially RFT. Yvonne is the cofounder of Perspectives Ireland and codeveloper of PBBT. She has 25 years of experience in behavior therapy.

Ciara McEnteggart

Occupation: Company Co-director of Perspectives Ireland

Dr. Ciara McEnteggart is a chartered behavioral psychologist with the Psychological Society of Ireland. She was a postdoctoral researcher at Ghent University from 2015 to 2020. Ciara graduated from the Department of Psychology at the National University of Ireland, Maynooth, in 2015 after completing an experimental Ph.D. in the application of RFT to complex behavioral problems. She has published one edited volume, over 40 scientific articles and book chapters, and given over 70 presentations and workshops internationally. Ciara is the cofounder of Perspectives Ireland and codeveloper of PBBT. She has 15 years of experience in behavior therapy.

Marjolein Vleugel

Occupation: Company director of Expertise Centrum ACT

Marjolein Vleugel (MSc) graduated from the University of Utrecht in 1998 with degrees in developmental psychology and clinical psychology. Since then, she has worked as a healthcare psychologist. As the owner of an ACT training facility in the Netherlands, she provides workshops for healthcare professionals, ACT therapy for individual clients, and has given multiple presentations about ACT. Marjolein has studied the clinical application of RFT in process-based therapy with Ciara McEnteggart and Yvonne Barnes-Holmes. As a member of the Association of contextual an behavioral science (ACBS), she has been on the board of the Belgium/Dutch Chapter.

Roy Thewissen

Occupation: Clinical Psychologist and behavioral Therapist

Dr. Roy Thewissen (PhD), who lives in Belgium, is a clinical psychologist and behavioral therapist. He works part-time at the pain department at the Adelante rehabilitation clinic in Hoensbroek (the Netherlands). Here, he introduced and helped shape the ACT model within the multidisciplinary group treatment. He supervises his team in adopting RFT principles in doing ACT with people with chronic pain and fatigue complaints. As a freelancer, he gives training, workshops, lectures, and supervision in experiential and process-based ACT, clinical RFT, and clinical behavior analysis. He is currently developing experiential and process-based ACT, informed by RFT, for the treatment of people with chronic pain and other somatic complaints.

Foreword

Standing at the cradle of art and science

Robyn D. Walser

As it turns out, a life well lived can be found in engaging in a few simple behaviors. If we move through the world with a sense of discovery, curiosity, and presence, we might better discern our meaning and purpose. Nonetheless, the simplicity of these behaviors is hard to engage and maintain. Us humans have an incredible capacity to sink into rigid places, caging ourselves before we ever open fully to our worlds. What is this cage? It is the very thing you are doing right now by reading this passage. It is language. Our relationship to our verbal selves, or our minds, gives us the unique capacity to stretch into life fully and purposefully. At the same time, it also has the capacity to hold us hostage to stories, thoughts, evaluations, and judgments about ourselves.

As a clinical psychologist, I have seen the joy of openness and the pain of rigidity. Clients in session have laughed and cried, feared, and calmed. They have experienced devastation, trauma, broken hearts, death, and loss of meaning. But they have also felt awe, pride, and wonder. They have overcome, facing barriers in the service of creating opportunities for change and growth. In each, I have seen the desire for love and connection, the desire to be accepted as whole and capable. Yet, they suffer under the veil of the mind and its sometimes painful offerings.

Through the work of acceptance and commitment therapy (ACT), I have seen true and lasting change. It is with some humility that I make such a claim, but I should clarify. Human suffering is not always easy to approach and overcome, especially since many in the world would suggest that overcoming pain means living inside of peace and happiness. I fully welcome each of these experiences, but also recognize that life holds its own measure of heartache and loss. Simply thinking good thoughts and having pleasant feelings cannot combat the nature of these experiences. We need a deeper understanding of what it means to be conscious beings who encounter a sometimes unfriendly world, a sometimes scary world, and a sometimes lonely world. We need a way to see ourselves fully without letting what we see lead us to run, hide, and fight, or corner us in the dark shadows of small and fearful living. Awareness to experience while choosing a broad and values-based life is why I say it is through the work of ACT that I see true and lasting change. It offers conscious living with choice and meaning.

Opening to the recognition that pain is part of what it means to be alive and meeting it with awareness allows a different relationship with our internal experience to unfold. If we no longer shrink away from pain, we might see that it is a part of life and that it holds vital, fundamental messages, should we choose to listen. These are messages of love and caring, messages of meaning. It is in this very pain that purpose is born. This sense of meaning and purpose is buoyed by the notion that we are more than our internal experiences, that we are beings who are thinking, feeling, and sensing dynamically and fluidly. We are in motion at all levels of our being; thus, no experience is permanent, nor is it the definer of who we are or must be. Possibilities emerge; freedom lives here.

Translating this open and aware approach to human suffering from an ACT perspective requires a commitment to understanding its nuances and a coherent theoretical approach linked to science, as well as a stance of compassion and humility. In their book, *ACT with Head and Heart: Working Process-Based with Acceptance and Commitment Therapy,* Lieve Bruyninx, Yvonne Barnes-Holmes, Ciara McEnteggart, Marjolein Vleugel, and Roy Thewissen offer a valuable path for clinicians to bring ACT alive in at least two forms: head and heart. Albert Einstein once wrote about the beautiful experience of mystery, noting its twofold gift: standing at the cradle of true art and true science. *ACT with Head and Heart* also offers this experience.

From key assumptions to case analysis to experiential work and relational frame theory, these five authors have created a book for clinicians that will guide them through the processes in ACT while providing foundational skills. The stance of an ACT therapist is not only described but also captured and transmitted in the text in relatable and heartfelt ways. The authors also dare to take a stance on creative hopelessness, a process for undermining control, declaring it a key aspect of the intervention. If we are to create the grounds of freedom for our clients in therapy, then letting go of control will be essential. I fully agree and hold that if we are to move in meaningful ways in our lives, then control of pain will not do; it steals freedom.

The authors anchor a sense of self by moving clinicians through the process of creating psychological space, making room for all that humans feel and encounter on the inside. This most fundamental aspect of ACT, the vast sense of self as experiencer, is explored in helping clinicians assist clients in acknowledging their presence and their sense of I-here-now. This sense of self is then linked to values-based living, engaging in full and purposeful behavior that instantiates meaning. In this work, I believe a life well-lived – a life of discovery, curiosity, and presence – is found.

Ultimately, the goal of *ACT with Head and Heart* is to provide clinicians with a gift that pays itself forward, not just in its clinical acumen but also in its link to science. It is a gift translated from clinician to client that will help both see the value in recognizing what it means to be human and what it means to taste all that life has to offer – the joy and the pain. It is a gift that helps clinicians and thus clients to see the ongoing flow of life, its rise and fall, noticing that the very thing we run from is the same thing we need – pain – so that we might also have joy. The authors stand at the cradle of art and science in *ACT with Head and Heart*. I invite you to do the same.

Robyn D. Walser, PhD, is the author of *The Heart of ACT* and coauthor of *Learning ACT*, 2nd Edition, and *The Mindful Couple*. She is an assistant professor at the University of California, Berkeley.

Introduction

Lieve Bruyninx

The first book on acceptance and commitment therapy (ACT) was published in 1999 (Hayes et al., 1999). Since then, ACT has become widespread and is increasingly used by care providers for a growing array of problems. Internationally, ACT is regarded as an evidence-based treatment for, among other things, chronic pain, depression, mixed anxiety, obsessive-compulsive disorder, addiction, binge eating, and psychosis. In addition, ACT is also used for broader life issues that do not necessarily meet diagnosis criteria. ACT is truly a transdiagnostic approach.

In essence, ACT is an experiential form of behavioral therapy that relies on a novel behavioral approach to language and complex cognition, relational frame theory (RFT). Language and all its implications are central to ACT. Over the years, RFT research has developed concurrently with ACT, but not always in parallel with ACT. Sometimes practitioners struggle to relate to the theory and to its use in their clinical practice.

In this book, we aim to reconnect ACT with its behavioral roots and with the central basic concepts of RFT. In our experience, behavioral therapists and other practitioners who work with ACT increasingly base their interventions on protocolized versions of ACT, rather than on an understanding of its underlying behavioral processes. As a result, the order and form of the exercises and metaphors sometimes become more important than the function they serve for clients in the contexts in which they are used. This can have a detrimental impact on the relationship with the client and, ultimately, on treatment effectiveness.

When the focus shifts from protocol to the individual clients and their contexts, work can be more readily tailored to the specificities of each individual client. At heart, ACT considers that the functions of clients' behavior can only be truly understood from the perspective of each client's particular context. In essence, a deeper understanding of the rationale behind an individual client's behavior could allow you to tailor your interventions to the specific circumstances of the client in front of you, aligning the function of your intervention directly with what this client needs. It will also help you to have a more precise sense of what you are doing and what you are targeting in your interventions and why.

A shift toward a clearer "behavior-in-context" perspective can potentialize your ACT work. It will improve the relationship with your clients because such a focus

DOI: 10.4324/9781032699691-1

will naturally make you ask more questions about how your clients see them-selves and the world. It will also ensure that your clients feel more seen and more profoundly validated. Finally, it will help you respond more quickly and make on-the-fly adjustments if a client does not respond to a metaphor or exercise as expected.

In this book, we'll present a flexible use of all ACT components based on a behavioral principle-based analysis of the context and function of the broad ar-ray of clients' behaviors, both in and out of the therapy room. We'll present how an integration of the relevant basic concepts of behavioral science and shared humanity is central to ACT and together constitute the head and heart of ACT, respectively.

Another important emphasis in this book is the centrality of experiential work and self-care for therapists. Thus, all chapters are set up in such a way that you can first personally experience the impact of exercises and interventions. In this, our purpose is threefold: (1) Let you experience for yourself what you ask of clients. (2) Offer you, as a practitioner exposed to human suffering, the care and attention you deserve. (3) Help you, when considering your next move, recognize what discomfort belongs to your clients and what discomfort stems from your own history.

The first chapter presents the theoretical knowledge necessary before you start your first ACT conversation with a client. We based this chapter on our experience of the importance for clinicians of linking these concepts as directly as possible to clinical practice.

Subsequent chapters then elaborate on the seven key components of ACT in a practical way, with many exercises and examples stemming from our own experi-ence. Anyone who has previously read an ACT book will notice that we have cho-sen not to present these components in the form of the classic "hexaflex." Instead, we chose to start with those components that are closest and most central to what we do in our own clinical conversations. For that reason, for example, self-as-content and self-as-context have been separated into two different chapters.

You will notice that there is a logical structure in the chapters. It is there for didactic reasons and also because we think that, for example, it is often the case that therapy starts with self-as-content work. However, that doesn't mean that's always the case or that we always follow the order set out in the book in our clinical conversations. We also don't conduct therapy like we write books: one component at a time. There is much more variability in our clinical conversations, using bits and pieces from each component when we need them. It is therefore important that you allow yourself to 'browse' through the different chapters according to your client's needs.

If using the hexaflex as a guide doesn't always deliver what you hope or your exercises don't move what you expect and you want to change that, this book is for you. The book is intended for mental healthcare professionals who want to understand why their clients do what they do and want to base their interventions on that. Thus, you can pick up this book either as a beginner in ACT or as someone who is more advanced. What you'll get are the basic scientific concepts and the components of the psychological flexibility model viewed functionally, interwoven with our own experiences and exercises to do yourself. In principle, you do not need any prior knowledge of ACT or RFT to benefit from reading this book. However, because this book integrates all aspects of working with ACT, we can imagine that some people may find it more comfortable to learn about the elements separately first.

We wish you a lot of fun reading this book!

Reference

Hayes, S. C, Strosahl, K. D., & Wilson, K. (1999). Acceptance and commitment therapy: An experiential approach to behavior change. New York: Guilford Press.

Chapter 1

What you need to know about connecting the heart of ACT with the head of ACT

Lieve Bruyninx

This book is about integrating the relevant basic concepts of behavioral science with the humanity that is at the center of acceptance and commitment therapy (ACT) – this is what we mean with the distinction between the head and the heart of ACT, respectively. This chapter is intended to create a starting point for this integration of head and heart across two parts. Part 1 presents a brief summary of the concepts of the basic behavioral science that you will need for this integration as it applies to your clinical work. I have tried to limit the amount of abstract material presented, so that you have what you will need for clinical application, but no more. Part 2 then offers an introduction to the essential elements of ACT, each of which is expanded in the individual chapters that follow.

There are two currents that run through this book and the clinical work with which it connects:

1. You will see that some specific concepts in behavioral science directly influence our clinical work, while other concepts may be relevant but their role in clinical practice is not as obvious. In a nutshell, we lean most heavily on the concepts of relational frame theory (RFT).
2. We recognize that in all types of therapy, it is difficult to keep scientific concepts directly connected with clinical interventions, and clinicians often struggle with a sense of disjoin between these two sides. However, a key aim of this book is to demonstrate that working connections between ACT and behavioral science are possible, and we offer many examples of what this looks like in practice. In short, we want to show you how to stay clinical and practical without losing the science.

Key starting assumptions when learning ACT

In order to facilitate these two currents, and to show you how to integrate your ACT practice with the concepts of behavioral science, there are a number of key starting assumptions that need to be embraced as you start out.

DOI: 10.4324/9781032699691-2

1. ACT emerged from the behavior therapy tradition. This means that your clinical focus should be on *behavior* – your behavior and the behavior of the client.
2. ACT assesses the behavior of human beings within their *history*. This follows from the assumption that every behavior happens in a *context* that is broader than current events.
3. ACT prefers to talk about emotional distress in the broad terms of *psychological suffering*. This preference highlights the view that *all* human beings experience considerable psychological pain at some point in their lives.
4. ACT is delivered in all contexts through deeply humane, respectful, and often painful interactions. Transformative therapeutic change is best facilitated when both the client and the therapist are able to fully engage in this journey. It is, thus, crucial that therapists have adequate training and experiential competence to manage these complex interactions.

Part 1: the head of ACT

My first encounter with RFT was a painful and confusing experience, and I still find some of the published material on the theory too complex and abstract. I would go as far as saying that trying to get my head around some of the concepts was at times overwhelming, and any connection of this material to my clinical work escaped me for some time. But across time and trainings, some concepts really landed for me and slowly found a way into my session plans and my interactions with clients. These are the core ideas I have presented below. In a nutshell, these were the big shifts that I experienced in going from the way I used to do ACT to the way I do ACT now.

Part 1 presents a brief summary of the concepts of the basic behavioral science, including RFT, that you need for the integration of ACT's head and heart in your clinical work. I have tried to limit the abstract material included in order to give you what you need and no more. The sections below, therefore, contain the items of knowledge that you should wrestle with before you start your first ACT conversation with a client. These consist of: (1) context surrounds all behavior; (2) let successful working be your guide as a therapist; (3) everything we do is behavior; (4) we exist through language; and (5) the functions of behavior matter most.

Context surrounds all behavior

You will often hear the odd-sounding phrase "act-in-context" in ACT circles. This comes from the philosophical worldview called Functional Contextualism, where there is a surprisingly broad definition of context. What helps me to appreciate this breadth is when I think about context as a 360° photograph, something that surrounds behavior at every level, including my own behavior at any moment. Of course, context includes what is happening directly in the immediate environment, such as time of day, level of heating in the room, how your body feels, and so on. At a higher level, context also includes, for example, those who live in your house with you, your income, and your socioeconomic status. But in Functional Contextualism and in behavioral science, context also includes history. And this definition of history is also extremely broad and goes back the whole way through evolution. In short, context is every current and historical layer that surrounds all of our behavior now and our behavior then (past and future). In line with these broad definitions of context and history, a core assumption in ACT is that behavior cannot be fully understood without at least incorporating some understanding of its context.

A key part of what shifted for me as a therapist when I began to appreciate the breadth and influence of context was the implications of this view for understanding individual behavior. Consider the following example: Imagine visiting your in-laws for the first time, and they refer to your partner by the name "little mouse." That would sound particularly strange to you because you know your partner as the confident adult woman she is now, and "little mouse" does not know her at all. However, you immediately begin to realize that your partner acquired this pet name because she was a very timid child, and as such, the name matched who she was then. Until you are made aware of this history and its strong contrast with your partner as she is now, it would be very difficult to understand how she could be referred to in this way. The point here is that hearing this childhood pet name gives you an insight into who your partner used to be and how she has changed across time. As a result, appreciating the historical context of her life deepens your understanding about why she is the way she is now.

What seems ironic about having such a broad view of context is that understanding a client's behavior as part of the very extended context of their lives and history feels a little like looking for a needle in a haystack. And yet, the reassuring fact is that the way to understand the client *always* lies in the context. Your job as a therapist is just to start looking in the most helpful place. Much of our clinical work is, in essence, an attempt to get an eye on the contextual information that is influencing behavior, rather like putting together a jigsaw puzzle. Imagine a client says to me, "I just don't understand people around me." I might search for more details with the follow-up question, "Do you mean you don't understand *everyone*, or is there someone in particular that you really find hard to understand?" This question helps me to gain more detail about the context in which other people leave the client feeling confused. Ultimately, the more I know about the context of their lives, the more I can decipher which aspects of context exert the most influence on the client's behavior. Then I can help to manage or change that influence.

Let successful working be your guide as a therapist

A key feature of Functional Contextualism that struck me immediately and was totally different from what I had learned before was the emphasis on successful working as a modus operandi. I had been classically trained as a psychologist to try to decipher what was "real" from what was "not real" in terms of understanding a client's experience. For example, my training taught me that from the perspective of the therapist, a client's delusion is not real, but from the client's perspective, the delusion *is* real. I was instructed that this difference was important and that, in this example, the therapist held the *correct* view of reality while the client held the *wrong* view. What I learned in successful working was basically opposite to this. I learned that setting goals and aligning my behavior with those goals is a more effective way of working as a therapist than struggling with what is or isn't real (in an ontological sense) and whose perspective this is from. I only realized later on that this way of operating comes from pragmatism and is the backbone of behavioral science.

What this new pragmatic way of thinking really did was to help me to set out therapeutic goals in a simple and clean way, and then to keep checking if my behavior in and across sessions stayed on that path. I found the simplicity and guidance of this incredibly helpful in my professional and personal life. I found it very appealing to not start with the view that clients had *gotten things wrong* and that my job was to make them see the light of reality. Similarly, it was of great comfort when I was struggling in my personal life to remind myself that I was not doing things *the wrong way,* but instead that at some level this way had worked up to this point. I felt there was much more respect in just starting with the view that the way the client is operating makes sense to them but is ultimately not working in the service of their happiness and fulfillment. I actually get more curious when I think that my job is to figure out how a client's life is operating and how I can help them make that operate better.

For me, there was another refreshing part of the pragmatic way of thinking that involved the freedom to choose successful working as one way of working, rather than believing that there was really *only* one way of working and that way was the *right* way. Successful working allows for an individual or therapist to choose the way of working that appeals to them the most, and of course, that leaves room for a therapist to choose *not* to be guided by successful working but to choose some other path. Essentially, what Functional Contextualism does is offer successful working as a way of operating that you can choose to guide your behavior or not. Again, feeling as if I had been set free from what was right versus wrong was liberating for me.

Successful working is at the very root of ACT as a therapeutic regime. Most of the techniques and exercises used in ACT are part of a shared therapist–client journey in which our job as therapists is to help clients realize that their system, as it stands, is not working for them and is, in many ways, working against them. I have often seen therapists wrestling with a client's perspective as right versus wrong or real versus unreal, and I have simply learned that the best way to do ACT is to situate it in successful working. In my experience, ACT techniques work their best if you focus on their workability. In a nutshell, a therapist can use ACT techniques as part of a therapeutic strategy that focuses on changing behavior that is wrong to behavior that is right, or changing unreal experience to real experience, but in essence, that wouldn't be doing ACT, or at least not doing it in the pragmatic, workable way it was designed.

Everything we do is behavior

In my professional training, I learned to categorize psychological experiences as different from each other, typically based on whether they occurred inside or outside the skin. Specifically, thoughts and emotions were categorized as mental, internal experiences, while behavior was everything else that you did on the outside. Even early on, this didn't make complete sense to me, and I had already come across key clinical examples that could not be differentiated in this way. For example, rumination was described as a pattern of thinking, but at the same time it was denoted as behavior. Nonetheless, it came as a huge revelation to me to learn that for behavioral science, everything is behavior, including thoughts, emotions, memories, sensations, and so on. However, consistent with successful working and a pragmatic perspective, the point here is that categorizing all of these events as behavior is believed to offer an effective means of predicting and influencing that behavior; it is not an argument that these events are behavior in an ontological sense. It took me a long time to switch from seeing feeling as an emotion to seeing it as a type of behavior and to realizing that the barrier between inside and outside the skin had much less influence on a person's behavior than I had previously believed.

When I fully wrestled with the view that the skin boundary was less of a boundary in functional-analytic terms than I had thought, my understanding of experiences like thoughts and feelings really expanded. For me, thoughts and feelings were no longer reasons *behind* behavior; they *were* behaviors that I could examine in their own right. This really helped me to see that thoughts and feelings are just parts of a system on the inside, just like action is a part of the same system on the outside, and their expression is part of the way that system is operating at that time.

In categorizing internal experiences as behavior, I was more able to appreciate that some types of behavior can be readily tied to context (you can easily see how context and that behavior interact), while other types of behavior cannot. For example, it is easy to see that your puppy gets excited and jumps around (behavior) when you put your sneakers on to go for a walk (context). But it is hard to see how to connect mood changes (behavior) or a lack of willingness to exercise (lack of behavior) to anything that is happening around you (context). Being able to see that some behavior–context interactions were more traceable than others helped prepare me for when I encountered RFT and its strong differentiation between the complex verbal behavior that we see in adult humans and the simple non-verbal behavior that we see in non-humans and young infants. In summary, although what we do as adults is hugely complex and hard to see, it is still just a type of behavior.

We exist through language

I have had many exposures to RFT concepts, but I learned most about the theory during clinical supervision, where the concepts were applied, rather than being understood in an abstract way. What I have tried to do in this section is to keep the relevant concepts to their most basic. Hopefully, throughout this book, you will learn to appreciate the power and utility of RFT concepts without getting over-whelmed by their abstractness and the decades of scientific thinking on which they are based.

In line with the view of everything as behavior, it was not a shock for me to learn that RFT uses the phrase "verbal behavior" synonymously with the words "lan-guage" and "cognition." Put simply, language and thinking are the same behav-ior. I have to remind myself regularly that language here does not mean speaking, although speaking is part of the way language works. Again, the pragmatism and successful working on which RFT is based do not force you to see complex psy-chological events as verbal behavior; they just offer this as a useful way to think of those events and to find ways to change them in a clinical context.

The basic idea in RFT is a surprisingly simple one – language allows us to put random stimuli together in various ways. For RFT, this is the behavior of relating, and the simplest form of this behavior is giving an object a name. For instance, you learn that a ball is called the word "ball," and by reverse, you learn that the word "ball" refers to, or means the same as, an actual ball. This simple naming skill is the first step in language as relating, and as we move through childhood, we are able to show different types of relating involving increasing numbers of stimuli. Let's work through a few examples to help you see different patterns of relating. Imagine as a young child that you learned that the word "teddy" means an actual teddy; this is called a *coordination* relation because you learned that the two stimuli (the word and the object) mean the same thing. You also learned that "dogs" are differ-ent from "cats"; this is called a *distinction* relation because you learned that these two-word stimuli do *not* mean the same thing and that each word is coordinated with a different object. Then you may have learned that "trucks" travel faster than "horses"; this is a *comparison* relation because you learned that in the relating of these two stimuli, one of them is greater in speed than the other (a more-than rela-tion). Around the same time, you learned that "day" is the opposite of "night"; that is an *opposition* relation. Later on, you would have learned that your mother is the daughter of your grandmother. This is a *hierarchical* relation in which your grand-mother is related to your mother as above her in terms of age (and your mother is below your grandmother); your mother is related to you as above you (and you are below her); and your grandmother is related to you as above you (and you are below her). It is immediately clear how hierarchical relations are more complex than other relations.

Throughout our childhood and adolescence, these relating skills get practiced over and over every day, with new stimuli, especially words, being related to other new stimuli all the time. This becomes the fabric of our lives as we become language-based. Indeed, relating becomes automatic, and soon we cannot even see ourselves relating stimuli together. But it is happening all the time, and by ado-lescence, you will be well practiced even at relating stimuli to "you," which is referred to as *deictic* relating. For example, you might relate others to you as better than you, and this relational response might influence numerous aspects of your behavior. All of these patterns of relating are just how language works as a system of knowledge and communication. What is most important to appreciate is that you cannot see that this is relating or the behavior it controls are occurring all the time. This is, of course, a sad state of affairs, but according to RFT, it is unfortunately an essential part of the way normal language develops, through which patterns of relating are established and fixed.

The functions of behavior matter most

When you first grapple with the core idea in behavioral science that everything you do is behavior, whether it is inside or outside the skin, it makes immediate sense that behavior simply cannot be random but must operate for some purpose. In other words, behavior must get established, must be maintained, or must cease to occur for reasons; otherwise, behavior would be just chaos, and that doesn't seem to be the case.

In behavioral science, every behavior has a function that connects the organism (you) to the environment in some way. This doesn't mean that that behavior is good or makes the organism happy; it just means that the behavior serves some purpose. For example, if your young son cries when he falls over, his behavior of crying serves the function of attracting your immediate attention and eliciting help. In this way, you can see that although crying isn't a nice thing to happen, it nonetheless serves the important purpose of enabling the child to get attention and help. This is not the same as saying that help is what he really wants (although that may be true); this way of talking just explains why he cries at that specific time, and this helps us to understand what the behavior leads to: attention and help. And of course, if attention and help follow, then his crying is reinforced, and it is very likely to happen again. Now imagine that at some point he cries for attention when he hasn't fallen, and you again attend to and soothe him. As a result, crying to get attention without falling has now been reinforced, and it is more likely to happen again. This is just how behavior works, and the most important part of the behavior in this example is not the crying itself but the fact that your son has learned that his crying evokes your attention. Thus, the function of crying here is to seek attention, and that is the learning pattern that you have established.

As the behavior of relating, language works in a similar way to the crying example above; language behavior has functions too. Let's look at a simple example. You learn to coordinate dogs with biting (dogs=biting) and biting with danger (biting = danger), and thus you coordinate dogs with danger (dogs = danger). For you, the purpose of this relating behavior is that you learn to predict that some dogs will bite you, and thus you learn to avoid them. This is an important piece of learning through meaning (dogs mean danger) because it teaches you to prevent getting bitten rather than having to be bitten first and learn afterwards. Another important element in this learning is that you learn that "danger" makes you feel afraid, and as such, one of the functions that gets established with the word "danger" is that it serves to elicit fear in some circumstances. Then, when you coordinate dogs and danger, the fear function of danger gets attached to dogs (dogs = danger = fear).

Let's look at another example, just to help you really see the purposes served by the behavior of meaning as relating. Imagine that I tell a child not to touch the oven because it is hot. The child will now coordinate the oven with hot, and both stimuli (hot and oven) will have the function of avoiding touching for that child. But "hot" likely also has a fear function, such that you get frightened if you think you are near something that is hot. Feeling fear in this case is an approach or appetitive function. So, when the child avoids touching the oven, that's an avoidance function, and when the child feels afraid around the oven, that's an approach function. Both have been established with the words "danger" and "hot" in some contexts. The notion of avoidance and approach functions will be elaborated on in subsequent chapters.

Part 2: the heart of ACT

Part 2, the heart of ACT, comes more naturally to me than the head of ACT, as described above. The first time I really felt the intensity of experiencing ACT for myself, it just felt right, like a place I was always meant to be. During my psychology education and behavioral therapy training, especially, I always had the sense that something was lacking. Now I know what that was. I was looking for more common humanity and less fixing of the "abnormal" than what I learned and experienced in those contexts. In the sections below, I have tried to summarize the three key parts of ACT that represent, for me, the very essence of its humanity and power. These consist of: (1) psychological suffering is normal; (2) experiential work is essential; and (3) the therapeutic relationship is the cornerstone.

Psychological suffering is normal

Like all psychologists, I received training in psycho-diagnostic work involving standardized questionnaires and psychometric instruments in order to label and diagnose clients. Essentially, this was training in the "what" of behavior, in terms of labeling what clients do. Thereafter, my postgraduate training in behavioral therapy was more about the "why" of behavior, in terms of asking why do clients engage in the behavior that we see. This latter question was far more interesting and helpful to my therapeutic work because, ultimately, my job as a clinician was to change behavior and not just describe it. What jumped out first for me in learning ACT was that labeling behavior in the traditional diagnostic or syndromal way that psychology does actually fails to recognize the normality of psychological suffering, which was, in fact, consistent with RFT's account of language.

The number of people who suffer from a labeled pathology at some point in their lives is so high that any division between normal psychology and abnormal psychology doesn't seem to make sense to me. We have all had family, friends, and colleagues who have experienced serious psychological pain, and if we are honest, most of us have too. In fact, I know more people who have suffered than I know who have not, which convinces me that psychological suffering is more normal than abnormal. At the same time, I understand why the history of psychology created a strong dividing line between normal and abnormal, because that was the traditional way of describing and explaining mental pain. In previous decades, mental pain was also talked about a lot less than today, and so it was easier to believe that less people suffered on the whole.

It therefore resonated deeply with me when I learned that ACT operates on the assumption (again based on RFT) that psychological suffering is normal and that, as a result, human happiness would be hard to achieve. That is, it is normal to suffer psychological pain, and this suffering is a direct consequence of our ability to use language, combined with external experiences in the world. When I teach ACT, I often remind the audience that babies and animals don't try to commit suicide. They feel pain and react to it, but this reaction does not include future plans to end their own existence. This capacity to look to the future in order to find relief from the present is a type of deictic relational responding using temporal relations (me-there-then as different from me-here-now), which allows us to plan for our holidays but also to contemplate suicide. There is just no evidence that pre-verbal infants or animals do this, but sadly, humans do it very often.

It seems important to acknowledge here that the assumption of suffering as normality does not sit comfortably with everyone. It is painful to think that one day you may experience psychological pain, if you have not done so already. Equally, it is frustrating to think that the psychological pain you have suffered is just normal and perhaps not unique or special to your situation. The key message in ACT is that psychological suffering is a normal, shared human condition and that it may not be helpful for clients or for your clinical work to hold onto the view that psychological suffering is abnormal.

Experiential work is essential

Experiential work has been a continuous feature of my working and personal life with ACT. In my first ACT conferences, I always chose experiential over knowledge-based workshops. Although this was a choice based on personal priorities at that time, I realize now that this helped me to experience ACT from the inside or from the client's side. Often, those experiences were deeply painful, but they helped me to see again and again why my behavior and my life got stuck, and why I made decisions that turned out to be hurtful to me or to the people I love. Experiential work offers the therapists a unique perspective on their own experiences in a safe environment, a combination that I believe is at the very core of ACT. In other words, as a therapist, you learn about your professional craft at the same time as you learn about yourself as a human being. Doing personal work before or during your work as a therapist in ACT has numerous advantages. Before I articulate these below, one thing seems important to emphasize: Whatever you do in ACT, no matter how painful, it will be worth it.

1. The first advantage, in my view, of personal development in ACT is that it will show you what obstacles are obstructing your view on your own behavior or on

the behavior of a client. We all carry a burden called hurt, a sore spot that can easily be scratched, perhaps by a client with a history that is similar to yours. If this happens (it does not mean you are a bad therapist or that you are doing ACT wrong), it will just be hard for you to stay emotionally present during those times. Experiential work for you in ACT won't prevent this from happening, but it will make it much more likely that you will see when it does happen, and you can then, for example, share that reaction with a colleague in an appropriate context. This will reduce the risk of you being reactive in the session.

2. Experiential work in ACT will teach you to distinguish between the details of your story and the details of a client's story. For example, many therapists struggle with trying to be amazing therapists or with trying to be helpful all of the time with a client. When this happens, the therapist might explain the need for these efforts by arguing that the client's behavior warrants them. But we have often observed that this type of behavior says more about the therapist's story than about the client's. That is, "having to help others," "being good enough," "being seen to be strong," and so on are all experiences and pressures with which therapists struggle. As above, these are best dealt with outside of sessions. The point here is that if you don't know the stories that own you, you'll never know for sure what some of your actions as a therapist are about.

3. Experiential work in ACT can serve the important role of 'regular maintenance for therapists' well-being'. Health care providers work in demanding job contexts that require them to focus primarily on the well-being of others, but with typically few resources or systems for the maintenance of their own well-being. Indeed, professional training in psychology almost universally prioritizes clients' well-being over therapists', which never made a lot of sense to me. As a result, it doesn't surprise me that professional burnout rates are high among mental health professionals (O'Connor et al., 2018). In professional trainings, we emphasize therapist 'self-care' and discuss how this can be shared regularly and in a structured way with appropriate colleagues. Our audiences are often surprised when we recommend this. It must be said that some organizations have good systems in place for exercising their duty of care to their therapists, but sadly, many do not. What is most surprising is that many therapists themselves only fully recognize the value of such systems after they have had a breakdown, burnout, or gotten to the point of professional exhaustion.

The therapeutic relationship is the cornerstone

In the last 20–30 years, clinical psychology has witnessed a seismic shift toward the use of therapeutic protocols. Sadly, my own trainings suggest to me that this shift has reduced the centrality of the therapeutic relationship. One of the issues that I encounter again and again in supervision and trainings is the need for therapists to get training in the therapeutic relationship. Although this relationship is a key foundation in most, if not all, therapies, it is at the very core of ACT, given the heavily experiential and transformative nature of that work.

The therapeutic relationship in ACT is the rock in which all of our clinical inter-actions are embedded. First and foremost, the relationship must offer a context of psychological safety that becomes increasingly conducive to the client exploring their own vulnerabilities and then choosing to share these with the therapist. I used the word "increasingly" here very specifically because it is a reasonable assump-tion that the client will not be able to express their vulnerabilities or their own sense of weakness to a stranger, let alone a professional, who in the client's view may live a life of more psychological strength and control. If you actually take a moment to think about it, you would likely admit that you would find it difficult to share your deepest secrets and weaknesses with a stranger, especially if you believed that your suffering was abnormal. In other words, all good relationships take time and effort to build, and the therapeutic relationship is no different. From this perspective, it makes little sense for the therapist to engage in explicit 'interventions' very early on while safety in the relationship is still being established.

The importance of building safety in the therapeutic relationship is keenly illus-trated by specific client groups and other aspects of individual clients. For example, many clients have difficulties with trusting others and painful histories of being invalidated by loved ones. In these cases, certain ACT techniques, such as defu-sion, have to be undertaken very carefully because distancing clients from their thoughts and feelings can easily be interpreted by clients as invalidation of those very experiences. When this is experienced by clients as them being made invis-ible, it will serve to reduce trust in you as a therapist, rather than to build trust.

Now consider a client who has a history of sexual violence perpetrated against her by male partners who now comes to therapy with a male therapist of approxi-mately her age. Although working closely with a trustworthy and supportive male therapist may be exactly what this client needs, it would understandably take her some time to be vulnerable to a male. Similarly, imagine a 55-year-old male CEO who comes into therapy with professional burnout and finds himself with a young female therapist. It is understandable that this client may feel that the therapist will be unable to really understand his experiences and pressures. In this context, the therapist will have extra work building credibility in their relationship if her ACT techniques are to work their best.

On the other hand, recall the point above about therapist's own stories influenc-ing their therapeutic work. Now imagine that a male therapist with a history of sex-ual trauma is working with a male client with a similar history. While this shared experience and similarities may enhance the bond between them, it may well offer fertile ground for the therapist's own blind spots and pitfalls. The main point here is that the therapeutic relationship must be made safe for both client and therapist before any intrusive and transformative therapeutic work begins.

At one level, it might not strike you as unusual that the client and therapist oper-ate as equals in the therapeutic relationship, but in ACT, this is a core working assumption, especially given the view that psychological suffering is normal. This was one of the most important revelations I had in ACT – that clients and thera-pists matter equally. Of course, the dynamics of therapeutic sessions prioritize the client's needs and struggles, but not because the client essentially matters more, but rather because this is the most workable way to create change in their behavior. This equality also helps therapists to manage the common sense of responsibility we have for changes in a client's behavior. Because ACT is so fundamentally based on choices, the choice to behave one way or another is always under the remit of the client, while the therapist is best viewed as the person who puts up the sign posts, which the client may or may not follow.

We also find in training that therapists feel that nothing is really happening in a session unless they are delivering some sort of intervention. This is very much at odds with ACT, where the relationship is a core part of the ongoing context, and as such, in a given session, perhaps all that is happening is that the relationship is being worked on and strengthened. Indeed, in supervision, when therapists are stuck, we often encourage them to dial sessions back up to the relationship and slow down or even stop trying to do interventions. This advice works almost every time because, as the therapist has become stuck in their interventions, typically the therapeutic relationship has also become stuck, and our advice allows this stuckness to be shared between the two parties and serves to remind them that all growth should emerge from the safety and support of that relationship.

Chapter summary and conclusions

This chapter was your first step on the journey toward integrating the heart of ACT with the head of ACT. Part 1 started with four key assumptions you need to be aware of before you start doing ACT. (1) Your clinical focus is on behavior. (2) Behavior is driven by our histories. (3) What clients present with is psychological suffering, rather than illness. (4) Therapists are first and foremost humane. Place these assumptions underneath your ACT work from the beginning, and the interventions and exercises you do will always come from the right place.

There is surprisingly little in behavioral science and RFT you need to wrestle with in order to do ACT, but some concepts from there do need to be fully understood for ACT to be properly anchored inside behavior therapy. Part 1 explored these concepts and what they really mean for your clinical work. The first concept you need to wrestle with is *context* because you need to understand the context surrounding behavior now and in the past if you are to understand that behavior. The second concept that should guide your ACT work is successful working. Setting goals and aligning your behavior with those goals will help to ensure that all your efforts are going in the direction you set out, and adjustments can be made on an ongoing basis where this is not happening. As a therapist, this can really set you free from judging a client's behavior as right versus wrong, but it also directs you and them more toward what is or isn't working. Perhaps one of the most difficult concepts in behavioral science to wrestle with is the concept of behavior itself, especially the fact that, for the wing of psychology, *everything* is behavior. Working from this perspective allows ACT clinicians to see thoughts and feelings as behavior in their own right.

What RFT brings specifically to ACT is its focus on complex behavior as language. For RFT, human behavior is about relating and the functions of behavior are in line with those relations. What this does for ACT is that it emphasizes that not only does all behavior have functions, but that these functions can only be fully understood if the relations to which they are attached are also understood. The fact that we see so much self-criticism and negativity in clients coming to therapy is readily accounted for in RFT by the meaning that emerges from relating arbitrary stimuli together and the fact that "you" can be one of those stimuli.

The first of the three core pieces of the heart of ACT is presented in Part 2, namely the view that psychological suffering is normal, emanates naturally from RFT, and highlights the ACT emphasis on human equality between therapists and clients (i.e., therapists suffer too because of the natural processes of language). This itself leads comfortably to the second core part of the heart of ACT, which emphasizes the need and rights of therapists to undertake experiential work for their own issues. There are many benefits of this feature of ACT for therapists' personal and professional lives, including minimizing the possible leakage of a therapist's personal difficulties into their client work. Given the need for both therapist and client to participate in moving and transformative experiences, it comes as no surprise that the therapeutic relationship is the third key feature if the heart of ACT and essentially the cornerstone of all ACT-based clinical interactions.

The approach I took in the current chapter was based on what I always wished for as a clinician – to combine what seemed important in the humanity of therapy with what science had to say. Basic behavioral concepts and RFT can seem overwhelming, but if you give them enough time and effort, you will see direct and significant benefits in your clinical work. It also becomes increasingly striking how well these concepts align with the more experiential heart of ACT. Indeed, rather than being antagonistic or incoherent with each other, the head of ACT (seen through the lens of behavioral science) and the heart of ACT (viewed as transformative experiential interactions between two equal persons) are two sides of the same coin.

Reference

O'Connor K, Muller Neff D, Pitman S. Burnout in mental health professionals: A systematic review and meta-analysis of prevalence and determinants. Eur Psychiatry. 2018 Sep; 53:74–99. doi: 10.1016/j.eurpsy.2018.06.003. Epub 2018 Jun 26. PMID: 29957371.

Chapter 2

Identifying and understanding client stories

Exploring self-as-content

Lieve Bruyninx

This chapter shows you how to explore the psychological story within which a client operates. In acceptance and commitment therapy (ACT), we use the term "story" to refer to the implicit narrative according to which a client lives, but of which they are largely unaware (at a fully conscious level). It is important to note that story does not refer to the actual narrative the client relays to the therapist. The various features of the story, including thoughts and feelings, are referred to as "self-as-content" because they are seen as the content of the story about the self, and these are a key focus in the early stages of therapy. It is better, therefore, to interpret self-as-content in a way that closely matches the phrase itself – the content of what clients think and feel about themselves (i.e., what self-based thoughts and feelings look like).

From an ACT perspective, the therapist's job regarding self-as-content may be summarized as follows: (1) To bring the main content pieces into the client's awareness and ongoing felt experience. (2) To bring the main content pieces into the therapeutic dialog. (3) To integrate that content into the broad self-story that has emerged through the client's history and show how that content came to control behavior as a result. (4) To increase awareness of the fact that allowing the story to control behavior has not worked well for the client's life thus far. (5) To distance the client, where necessary, from felt experiences that are inside the story but have been experientially avoided. (6) To use this distancing from specific content to facilitate acceptance of that content and its role in the self-story. (7) To change aspects of the content and/or primarily the behavior controlled by that content in a direction that is workable and aligned with what the client values. This chapter will deal primarily with Points 1 (bringing content into the client's awareness and ongoing experience); 2 (bringing content into the therapeutic dialog); and 3 (integrating content into the broad self-story and showing how content is unworkable), with the remaining points coming under the remit of subsequent chapters.

The current chapter contains a number of sections. Prior to grappling with the client's self-as-content, the first section shows you how to set the broad initial context for doing ACT with a client (or group). The sections thereafter unpack how the story is brought to the client's awareness and developed through the therapeutic dialog. These sections are as follows: (1) Unpacking the content pieces of the story.

DOI: 10.4324/9781032699691-3

(2) Seeing how self-as-content pieces work together. (3) The client's role in self-as-content. (4) Stepping outside of self-as-content. It is important to emphasize early on that it is notoriously difficult in ACT to separate one piece of therapeutic work from another, mostly for the reasons discussed in the previous chapter.

Case Erik: part 1

In the following chapters, we will add a short case description for each component. At the start of each chapter, we will briefly introduce the case, and by the end of the chapter, you'll be able to get a sense of how the component has been targeted for each clinical case.

The first case is Erik (58 years old). Erik opens our first conversation by telling me that this is the second time he's experiencing burnout. He says he went back to work too soon after his first burnout. Since then, he recounts how he has felt constantly on edge. Following his second crash, he has felt constantly rushed and utterly exhausted. He has been seeing a life-coach for a year, but feels he needs clearer direction and more guidance. He wants something that will actually help him move forward. Erik's request could be rephrased as follows: "I want to be able to relax more, I want to stop feeling so rushed, and I want to be able to take on tasks at a normal, relaxed pace."

Setting the context for ACT

In this section, we aim to give you the tools you need to provide the client with a safe working sense of what to expect from you and what is likely to be expected from them in return. The way you start therapy sets the context for many of the interactions that will occur between you and your client. Hence, it is important from the first encounter that your broad stance and your specific actions are ACT-consistent, and that the client has a reasonable sense of what these will be. For example, we typically inform clients that ACT may look and feel different from what they have encountered before, including discussing our view of the normality of psychological suffering (see Chapter 1). What we are trying to achieve at this point is a shared commitment between both parties on something we can work toward together initially and on something that can build up to more complex and challenging commitments later on. Although establishing these early aspects of therapy seems straightforward, it faces an immediate challenge in terms of the resistance clients bring to the first sessions.

It is hard to change the ways you've been trying to change. Although it seems ironic, at one level, all clients are initially resistant to certain changing aspects of their behavior. This is not because they really don't want to change or because they haven't tried hard enough. I have rarely seen a client who has not genuinely tried everything they knew to change what they do or who they are. It is not their efforts that are at fault, but the strategies through which their efforts are directed. Put simply, it is not that they haven't tried, but just that what they have tried hasn't worked (or they wouldn't be where they are). As a result, we heavily validated and normalized the genuine place from which their efforts emanated. Everyone loves a tryer, and clients are real tryers. Indeed, that is how we want them to stay throughout therapy. It's just that their trying will be turned in a totally different direction. So, the resistance we see in clients at the beginning of therapy is not general resistance to change, not at all, but it is more accurately described as resistance to trying to change in a completely different way. If we link this to the client's self-as-content, we would say that all of their efforts to change thus far have been from *inside* their story (content-based), and we will direct them toward change that is *outside* their story (context-based). In ACT, we actually go a step further than this and say that the most natural, sensible ways to solve problems can ironically contribute to the problems themselves. That is, what seemed like the solution until now has actually been part of the problem.

The change efforts clients describe at the beginning of therapy are typically rigid and rule-based (e.g., "you should never put yourself before others" or "you should never speak badly of the dead"). In other words, they tend to see what they have been doing (and themselves for doing it) as fundamentally wrong or stupid, rather than seeing what they have been doing as unworkable, ineffective, or rigid and inapplicable in certain contexts. What is important at this early stage is to help clients to notice these harsh judgments about themselves and about their change efforts and instead develop a sense of curiosity about their efforts and the work-ability of these efforts in terms of whether they have led to the desired outcomes or not. This feels much more curious than judgmental and permits more room to experience the frustration they typically feel because their efforts have not paid off. In order to validate their change efforts while recognizing that they have not worked and are still drawing the client toward a new way of operating, the therapist might say something like this.

When change efforts have not worked example

Many therapists work on changing how you actually think and feel, and that makes a lot of sense. But it seems to me that this basically describes what you have already tried, and you seemed to have tried really, really hard to change the thoughts and feelings that show up for you. But to be honest, that just doesn't seem to have worked, and I think there is a part of you that has a sense of that. So, maybe a different approach is worth looking at here. And maybe if we look at your situation a certain way, we might actually see that the way you've been trying to change, albeit admirable and honest, has become part of the problem and not part of any solution. And perhaps that is part of why you feel so tangled up with your troubles and so stuck with them.

Real change is going to be long and painful. It is somewhat ironic that although most clients have engaged in enormous efforts to change, they still feel that they are just missing something small, something critical that they need to figure out and remember, and when they do that, they will be able to stay on the right track most of the time thereafter. As a result, they come to a professional to get the right or best piece of advice, and then, according to their story, they will be able to follow that perfectly, and all will be well. This is the reason why ACT practitioners tend to be cautious about the widely held view that deep, lasting change can be achieved quickly. In practice, this is rarely the case. The part of this type of quick-fix thinking that is most unhelpful is that it ignores the reality that most clients have experienced very painful histories, day after day, and the impact of those histories that spanned years simply cannot easily be undone in 30 or even 50 one-hour sessions. Consider the generic example of a 50-year-old woman who was physically and emotionally abused by a parent every day until she ran away from home at 18. If we calculate that she spent 18 years of 365 days at home, and if we simply say that she experienced one hour of abuse every day (huge oversimplification), that makes a total of 6,570 hours of abuse. Now perhaps it's easier to see how little even 100 hours of therapy compares to this.

The other unhelpful aspect of quick-fix thinking is that it fails to fully wrestle with the fact that the path toward genuine freedom and mental wellness is a painful one. Specifically, when emotional avoidance begins to reduce, clients will actually experience the fullness of the pain that they have thus far avoided. In simple terms, at key points in ACT, clients will experience more felt pain than when they first come through your door. Because this too runs counter to what many clients initially believe, we make this an important part of the early dialog, using metaphors such as the one below (Hayes & McCurry, 1989).

Stirring up a dirty glass metaphor

What we will be doing in these first few sessions is like cleaning out a glass with water on the top and sand on the bottom. That's sort of the way you are now. At one level, you seem to be doing okay, but at another level, something heavy and dirty underneath seems to be weighing you down. But it probably won't surprise you to hear that some of what we will be doing in here is stirring up that sand. This means that the water will get dirty, and you'll naturally start to feel unsettled because we'll be unsettling the water by shaking the sand up through it. That's just part of what we might need to do to get a real sense of what all the various parts of you feel like and how they sit together right now.

Because a radical overhaul of change efforts is needed and because this will take huge commitment in terms of time and effort, among other things, it is essential early on to create a context where this commitment can be managed, valued, and given everything it needs to work. In practice, it is preferable to see all clients weekly and to have a commitment from both parties for an initial period of ten sessions and to review every week sessions thereafter. In our experience, not seeing new clients weekly slows progress down and can restrict the experiential aspects of ACT and the building of safety and intimacy that transformative therapy needs. The therapist might introduce this commitment using a metaphor like the one below.

Starting a new exercise regime metaphor

Early on, this will feel like starting a new exercise regime. It's hard at the start because everything seems new and confusing, and part of you will feel like you don't fully have a handle on it. And of course, a big part of new exercise is that it hurts. Parts of you (muscles) that you never even felt before start to hurt. And that can be frustrating because when you're working hard to move forward, it can actually feel like you're going backwards because you might even be feeling worse. But I suppose it's true when they say that progress hurts. Maybe that's even one of the ways in which we'll know we're progressing in here. And, if you are moving ahead, you will know it, and we will both see it in your life. It is just that we can't be sure of this on a week-to-week basis. So, to give this new regime the time and space it needs to become a real working thing, I would like us right here and now to make a solid commitment to it, at least in terms of time. Let's start with committing to ten sessions on a weekly basis. Could we commit to that right here and now in order to help us have an anchor in case you start to feel the pressure and really feel like you want to quit at some point? Of course, that happens a lot with new exercise regimes. I'm not saying that everything you want will be achieved by then. I'm just saying that by then, if it is helpful, you will know it, and we will both know we are heading in a good direction. Then, together, we can choose where to go from there based on where we have been between now and then.

Work at the client's pace. At the beginning of therapy, it can be difficult to have genuine respect for where a client is at, because they are so tangled up. However, without being drawn into too much detail, it is essential that the therapist begins just where the client is at and slowly, methodically works from there. I have seen therapists over and over who are keen to get things moving and act hastily, even if with good intentions. This actually makes the client feel that their struggles are being glossed over and sets a context that is the opposite of what you both really need. It is not surprising, therefore, that the questions we ask are not typical intake questions. And in my experience, when I have been required to conduct a standard intake interview, it actually gets in the way of seeing the content that is causing the problem because clients do their best to give you the content that answers your questions. It is important to find your own voice in this early part of therapy, and that takes practice. The following questions are examples of how you can get started in ACT.

Sample questions to move toward self-as content

- *I'm sure you have a lot of difficult stuff going on, so let's just start with the thing that has bothered you the most in the last couple of days, weeks, or even months.*
- *I'm sure there are several reasons why you came here, and lots of things you need to tell me, so if I could wave a magic wand right now and change one single thing about what you're feeling or thinking, what would you change first?*
- *I'm guessing that like all my other clients, you feel like there's a ton of things inside you that have been holding your life back from where you want it to go, could we start by you telling me some of the things that are really getting in your way of living.*
- *In terms of things that you think and feel very strongly or often, what would you say are your top three reasons for coming to see me?*

Unpacking the content pieces of the story

Because we are trying to detect various key pieces of self-as-content here, it helps to use a metaphor that highlights things that have pieces but which we typically perceive as one whole thing. This type of metaphor offers a gentle hint (which we will pick up on later in therapy) that the parts form a whole, and when we think about the whole, it makes it difficult to see the parts directly. We often use a metaphor about McDonald's for this. As well as opening up the idea that we all have content pieces, this metaphor presents the key idea that some pieces are perceived as positive, while others are perceived as negative.

The McDonald's metaphor

What's your favorite food at McDonald's? (Let's say it's a Big Mac). So, you just love the way Big Macs come out – all tall and juicy. They're just a perfect finished specimen when they're done and ready for you to eat. But it's funny to think about the cook who put it all together. They just went to the fridge and pulled out a cold slice of sticky meat. And then they lifted up a few slices of cold cheese. And then they reached in, got a bun, and sliced it. And then they got a piece of lettuce (and so on). And at one level, that's all a Big Mac is – just those few bits and pieces stuck together, like when they say the whole is more than the sum of its parts. And let's just think about each part. The piece of lettuce just on its own would probably be pretty horrible. And the bun on its own would be really plain. Even the meat wouldn't taste the same without the other pieces. So, what if I asked you about the smaller bits and pieces that show up in your mind that are all part of the story you live by. I guess there would some bits you could stomach on their own and some bits you really couldn't. Maybe you could think about one bit you would be happy to have on its own, and then one bit you definitely wouldn't want to have on its own.

Let your own experiential work guide you. In trying to understand a client's story and get a view of the key content pieces, we lean heavily on the experiential ACT work we have done in our own lives. This work on ourselves teaches us to take up a position outside the content of our own individual story and instead learn to use self-as-context as a place to anchor our mind and feet (see Chapter 7). We will refer regularly to these personal insights and experiences throughout this book, and in various parts of the text, we will encourage you to use yourself as a working example of the ACT techniques we are explaining. To help you do this, we have inserted empty text boxes, such as the one below, in which you can write when we ask you to reflect on specific things.

Let's do a simple personal exercise using the first text box below.

Exercise: introducing yourself

Imagine you and I were to meet in person, how would you introduce yourself to me? What are the first three key lines you would share with me about yourself?

Please write your answers here.
1.
2.
3.

Look carefully at what you wrote above and notice that, given the context, you probably provided cursory surface-level information, such as your name, your age, your profession, and so on. And if 20 or even 50 lines had been provided, you probably would still have provided that same type of neutral, even positive, information about yourself. The point here is that you are very unlikely to have written anything negative or painful about yourself in this context, no matter how many lines you had been given. We all want to make good first impressions, and we all want to believe that the positive pieces of content, more than the negative pieces, are more real and dominant in reflecting our worth as human beings.

If we think about all the neutral or positive pieces you wrote in the box above as the nice bits inside the Big Mac, now we'd like you to focus on the not-so-nice bits. Reread what you wrote slowly, and then think carefully about what you *didn't* write. Really think about what you normally wouldn't write. You probably didn't write that you sometimes judge yourself harshly, that you have made stupid mistakes, that you think you are lazy, and so on.

Exercise: three negative things

Would you now consider, in the privacy of this conversation with yourself, writing down some of these negative ingredients that go into your Big Mac? Would you be willing to write down below the three most negative things you regularly think about yourself?

Please write your answers here.
1.
2.
3.

Seeing how self-as-content pieces work together

Little or no self-as-content that is presented in therapy and causes distress is evaluated as neutral. What clients are juggling is a sense of stuckness between self-as-content that is positively evaluated and self-as-content that is negatively evaluated. We introduce this stuckness in The Ham Sandwich Metaphor.

The Ham sandwich metaphor

It seems to me when I listen to all the parts that you've been talking about that they might go together something like this. It's as if you are a prepackaged ham sandwich. On top, the bread looks inviting and makes you just want to bite into it. On the bottom, where no-one looks, the bread is soggy and wouldn't taste good at all. So, that's why it's at the bottom and definitely not at the top. And you're a bit like the ham squeezed between the two. You're stuck between the good things you think and feel about yourself at the top, and the bad things you think and feel about yourself at the bottom. And, of course, ham sticks. And naturally, the more it sticks to the bottom piece of bread, the more you want the ham to stick to the top piece. So, you do your best to stick to the top and not the bottom. But, either way, you're still trapped in between what you think and feel.

Let's talk metaphorically. Clients typically come in with a specific piece of negative content (e.g., feelings of anxiety) held tightly in one hand. They lay this down flat on the table, spread it all out in front of you, and say something like, "Look at how bad this is. Please fix this, so I can do better." Typical examples of highly believable pieces of self-as-content that are laid bare before you at the beginning of therapy are presented in the box below.

Examples of tightly held pieces of self-as-content

1. "*Anxiety* has taken over my life. I can't go to work or see my friends anymore because of it. I'm even too afraid to leave the house. It's ridiculous, I'm getting anxious over nothing, there must be something wrong with me."
2. "For now, I'm on sick leave because the *pain* has been so bad. I need to get back to work. I have responsibilities there and I can't keep being a burden to my colleagues. There's no reason why this pain just shouldn't go away, the doctors tell me there's nothing wrong."
3. "I'm just *numb*. I'm empty. Nothing means the same as it used to. I've just completely lost it and I don't think I can get it back. I can't explain how this all happened. If I keep this up, my partner just won't be able to take this anymore and then I'll really be in trouble."

It is entirely understandable why strong, recurring, and painful pieces of self-as-content (such as anxiety, pain, and emptiness) dominate the client's attention and form the basis of what they come into therapy with and plead with you to reduce or eliminate. I often use the common analogy of the most painful, recurring, or largest piece of this type of content as being the "straw that broke the camel's back," referring to the fact that this has now forced the client to seek professional help. In a nutshell, we want to explore this final straw, as well as all the other straws the camel is dealing with. In the box below, please write down any straws that you experience on a regular basis and any one in particular that you have felt has, or may eventually, break the camel's back.

Exercise: the straw that broke the camels back

Please write your answers here.
  Straw 1.
  Straw 2.
  Straw 3.
  The straw that might eventually break/has broken (delete as appropriate) the camel's back.

Let key content pieces emerge without trying to change them. In supervision, it emerges again and again that junior therapists have difficulty in sitting patiently as key pieces of self-as-content are emerging (another area where experiential work helps). Naturally, they "want to get to the bottom" of the story and then move it around with interventions. Indeed, this is a key area in which ACT is notably different from other therapeutic regimes. This part of therapy is slow, organic, and not heavily directive. Your job is essentially to see the key pieces of content shine through what the client says to you directly, just respect them, and gently begin to point them out as you see them from your perspective (preferably as another human being looking in and not primarily as a professional or therapist).

Although this early phase of therapy might feel pointless or slow, something very useful is actually happening. As key pieces of self-as-content are emerging, the client is learning to observe and talk about that content through the perspective of another human being (you), as different from the inward, confusing, stuck perspective within which content is normally experienced. In a nutshell, you are functioning as a safe, observant bystander. You are not overwhelmed by any piece of content, no matter how bad or painful, you can see it, notice it, and reflect it back gently to the client from where you are standing. This is a gentle but powerful shift in perspective-taking.

Although this part of therapy is non-directive in the sense that you have no desire to move content around, you have to find a way of ensuring that key content pieces rise to the surface of what the client tells you, and that can take some clever probing on your part. Typical examples of questions I ask for this purpose are presented below. You can see how they are a step further, and a little more intrusive, than the opening questions from before.

Sample questions to draw up key pieces of self-as-content

- *What you've just told me really touches me. I'm sure that was hard for you to say. So, if we could pick through that, which do you think is the most painful piece stuck inside there?*
- *It seems like there is a lot going on in your head and in your body, let's take our time and look closely at anything that really stands out above the rest?*
- *You seem to put a lot of emphasis on the fatigue, and I can see why, but what is it about it that really gets in the way or your life?*
- *If I turned up the volume inside your head or your chest, what would shout loudest or most often?*

The questions you ask at this point need to direct the client's attention to certain parts of what they are telling you. You are asking about details, but not because you need all of them, but rather because you are trying to understand why those details matter in the way that they do to that client. You will see in the mini-transcript below how these questions are presented. It should look less like "Please tell me more about this detail" and more like "What do you think this really means?"

In the interaction below, it becomes clear that "making mistakes" means a lot more to this client than the mistakes themselves. Making mistakes appears to have

---

**Mini transcript on identifying pieces
of self-as-content**

Therapist: You just told me that you can't make mistakes. I wonder if we could explore what it's like for you as a person who can never make mistakes. For example, what has happened when you did make a mistake in the past, or what would happen if you made a mistake today or tomorrow?

Client: Everybody would get angry, and I wouldn't be able to cope with the conflict. The only choice I have is to work harder and act as if they can't touch me.

Therapist: So, you have to work really hard all the time to make sure that there's no anger or conflict? Is that what a lot of that hard work is about?

Client: I can't take the risk. Never. And, I have to be especially careful with my family. They have all these opinions about me and what I do.

Therapist: That sounds like a lot of very hard stuff to be trying to juggle all the time. But, I guess you just feel like you have to, and that it's really worth it, because the risks are too high if you don't?

Client: I don't have a choice. They can't know that I'm afraid. I have to stay strong all the time. If they knew I was really afraid, they could hurt me and they'd take advantage of that.

Therapist: So, if I peer into all the stuff you're talking about here as if it were a box, I would see: fear that you could get hurt; fear that you could get cut off from your family' maybe fear of loneliness; lack of choice; risk, conflict; and ultimately rejection and loneliness? That's a lot of bad stuff in one box.

---

powerful consequences that have to be avoided because mistakes carry a huge threat to her psychologically and even to the routine of her life. I would even go as far as saying that her fear of making mistakes is legitimized by a real sense of impending danger. In this case, we would say that threat, danger, and rejection are important pieces of self-as-content operating underneath making mistakes, and it is these pieces that our ongoing dialog is trying to identify.

The client's role in self-as-content

There is often a question in our trainings about why some pieces of self-as-content become more sticky than others. That is, some people struggle more with dread than fear, some with shame rather than guilt, and so on. Indeed, it is true that clients will vary considerably in this regard, but the one piece of the puzzle that spans all clients is that the content becomes problematic because they invest their behavior in it, usually in the function of avoidance. At the same time, there is a delicate balance to be struck here between recognizing the extent to which the client feels helpless or stuck and the fact that their own behavior is part of what keeps things the way they are. The way these two opposing forces are reconciled is to present it to the client that it is understandable that they simply cannot help doing what they are doing while things remain as they are. For example, we emphasize that the client is the helpless recipient of their own thoughts and feelings, and as such, they feel compelled to act when these show up. The theme you want to suggest in all of this is that the client is being pulled along, almost helplessly, and not genuinely able to exercise their own choice. This is not an issue of blame or responsibility; rather, it is establishing a context in which the client self-criticizes less and realizes that the force of their history has simply been stronger than them. The following mini transcript contains the lion-tamer metaphor, which is incredibly helpful at this point in therapy.

Mini transcript on identifying the client's role in content
(The lion-tamer metaphor)

Therapist   What's happening to you seems a bit like what goes on between a lion-tamer and the lion. The lion-tamer cracks the whip to tell the lion that they won't be happy if the lion doesn't perform, exactly the way he has been trained. So, the lion keeps performing, because it's afraid of the whip. And yet, there is a little piece of that lion that just wants to be free to roam, because roaming is what lions do.

Client: Are you saying that I'm afraid to do what I want because I think I would be punished?

Therapist: I think there is probably a bit of that in here. But, if we just focus on what's happening inside you, rather than what's happening outside, the situation inside too is like the interactions between the lion-tamer and the lion. What I mean is that there is a part of you that behaves like the lion-tamer, and there is also a part of you that has to be the lion.

Client: I never thought of it like that. So, you are saying I'm the one cracking the whip on myself?

Therapist: In a way, I am saying that. It just seems like your mind tells you that you have to keep performing; your fear tells you that you have to keep performing; and your anxiety tells you that you have to keep performing, and so on. So, just like the lion, your feet and hands keep performing. And yet, doesn't it ring true that there is a little part of you that just wants to be free from that whip?

Client: So, I shouldn't trust the lion-tamer, and I should listen to the little voice?

Therapist: You could start just with recognizing those parts of you that are the pushy lion-tamer and noticing the things they make you do.

Instructions from the lion-tamer exercise (1)

Please write down the five most common instructions your lion-tamer gives you. These probably include: work hard; be kinder; get healthier; get more attractive; earn more; achieve more; gain more knowledge; gain more insight; and so on.

1. *I* should...
2. I must...
3. I need to...
4. It is important that I...
5. I have to...

Instructions from the lion-tamer exercise (2)

Now write down the five most common actions that you engage in that try to deliver on these demands. These probably include: working hard; being kinder; trying to get healthier; putting yourself under pressure to achieve more; trying to look clever in front of others; and so on. Copy your original answers from above in the first, and then answer the second part of each. For example, if you wrote above "I should lose weight," then below you might write underneath that "I regularly start a new diet on Mondays."
    For example:
    When the lion-tamer says: "I should value my health more", then I go on a diet.

1. When the lion-tamer says I should...
    Then I ...
2. When the lion-tamer says I must...
    Then I ...
3. When the lion-tamer says I need to...
    Then I ...
4. When the lion-tamer says it is important that I...
    Then I ...
5. When the lion-tamer says I have to...
    Then I ...

The key ACT message at this stage in working with self-as-content is to fully appreciate the almost compulsive, can't-help-it way in which your actions follow your mind's instructions. It helps to think of this as investing more content in content. This passivity is genuine and says nothing at all about an individual's desire to change their behavior. In a nutshell, as therapists, we must completely let clients 'off-the-hook' for what they have been doing over and over to this point. They haven't done anything wrong or even anything foolish. They have simply done what the lion-tamer forced them to do, and now they are seeing their behavior as that for the first time. Ironically, this recognition gives space for change, without guilt or defense.

Same behavior, same outcome. As clients really get to grips with their ongoing behavioral investment in their content, and recognize this as a key obstacle to change, it takes several sessions for them to look carefully at the detail in their daily routines and see experientially how often they behave like a lion and how dominant the lion-tamer is, day after day. We often refer at this point to the movie Groundhog Day. However, there is an interesting twist here that therapists need to be alert to. An important piece of our repetitive behavioral patterns is that any change in topography, even when the function is exactly the same, convinces us that we are doing something different and that something different will happen as a result. In other words, we believe that we are engaging in new behavior that will lead to a new outcome. But in purely functional terms, the fact is that the behavior is the same, and thus the same outcome will inevitably follow.

This function-over-form focus is very important here because it brings clients to a place where they start to mistrust their own behavior because they cannot be sure anymore that they really are (functionally) different. This can be a despairing experience because it often brings with it a sense that "I'll never get this right," and that must be recognized. But what is more important is that the therapist encourages the client to metaphorically stand still. There is a common metaphor in ACT called the tug-of-war with the monster that describes the client pulling one end of a rope, and using the example above, we might say that the lion-tamer is on the other end. And what we are encouraging clients to do here is simply drop the rope. This is a very powerful move, and functionally speaking, it is also new because, for new behavior to start, sometimes old behavior needs to stop first. Indeed, to really emphasize this move, we often have clients visually imagine the rope and then imagine dropping it slowly, letting it fall inch by inch to the ground, never to be picked up again. A parallel benefit here is that the client feels a sense of self-efficacy and empowerment, albeit in a humble way, that counteracts to some extent that despondency about never being able to change, as noted above. This very act of dropping the rope in our physical metaphor opens up the possibility for a different outcome because, in and of itself, it is a new behavior. This simple metaphor can then be referred to again and again in coming sessions when clients revert back to content pieces and content-based actions, and the therapist can say things like "It looks like you have picked up the rope again" or "I think I see the rope sitting tightly in your hand as you speak." Another important thread that is being maintained here with the focus on behavior and consequences is that it keeps away from any sense that the problem is the client per se.

Stepping outside of self-as-content

Another key feature of the lion-tamer metaphor is that it hints toward the idea that although your thoughts and feelings are like the lion-tamer, and although your arms and legs are like the lion, there is another little piece of you in there somewhere that is watching all of this and doesn't like what they see. This is typically the first point at which we direct the client's attention toward a place that is beyond self-as-content. Doing so prior to this point risks the same behavior-same outcome problem in functional terms. Thus, it is intentional that the little voice is only a small part of the lion-tamer metaphor.

In my experience, even at the beginning of therapy, most clients have a deep sense that their lives could, or should, have been different, and this is what we are appealing to here. We might think of this as a little voice of the self that is often overruled but is now being recognized by the therapist. Indeed, we often use the analogy of the little inner voice that has been silently operating underneath the lion-tamer's loud demands. We typically say things here like, "Hasn't that little voice been saying all along that they want something different for this lion, something that isn't jumping to someone else's whip? Do you recognize that?" Our aim is to gradually teach the client to listen to her own reactions to her experience and use these as a new source of influence over behavior. However, there is an important caveat to be made here, as follows. It is easy to see how quiet inner voices can also be perceived as more of the same type of self-as-content that the client can struggle with. And that is indeed a risk we do not want to take, hence our extreme caution about when we present this inner voice piece. We often avoid this difficulty by using the analogy of the narrator, where the narrator is a completely neutral character who simply narrates on every detail of your life and, as such, describes all of the details of the content. As a result, the analogy places the narrator outside of the content, rather than inside it, thus avoiding the more content problem.

In my own life, I found that stepping outside my self-as-content and stepping into the narrator's shoes was one of the most difficult ACT moves of all. For me, it was easier to identify with the lion-tamer and even with the lion than to identify with the little voice that recognized there was something terribly wrong with living a life in the circus, because that was simply too painful a place to stand. While I fully recognize the irony of what I am saying, it remains true, at least for me, that I was more comfortable as the lion just doing what my content dictated because in there it seemed as if I was shielded in some way by the sadness of having lived a life I really never wanted. In other words, being in the narrator's shoes is a very painful place to be.

As an illustration, let's look at what you may be experiencing at this very moment as you are reading this text. Maybe you are having the thought that you don't really understand what ACT is. As that thought gets larger, you might get a tight feeling in your throat. Now, you are remembering that you often get that tight feeling in your throat when you find things hard, and you also remember that you get that feeling when you have the thought that you are failing at something. And now, just as the word "failing" has come to your mind, you're having another really fast thought, "Maybe, I am a failure"; now the thought, "What if I never get this"; and then the thought, "What if I am just not up to this job?" And you notice that your whole chest is tight now. And you feel like you are in the grip of something.

The critical point is this. Even as the narrator, you are actually experiencing painful, judgmental thoughts about yourself, and you are still having overwhelming feelings and sensations. That is, there is still self-as-content happening to you. It is tempting to secretly believe that stepping outside of the story as the narrator will loosen the intensity of our self-as-content. But, experientially, this is not the case at all. We think what we think when we think it. And, we feel what we feel when we feel it. That said, something slightly different is happening in functional terms. This is a key distinction in ACT that takes a long time to really wrestle with. When we move to the narrator's position outside of the story, we can begin to see that no matter what we think or feel, we may now be in a position not to use our arms and legs to do what that content tells us to do. In a sense, we have begun to separate the lion-tamer from the lion. As the narrator, we are just describing in detail everything the lion-tamer does, as well as everything the lion does in response. The narrator sees that every thought we have about ourselves is like the lion-tamer insulting us. The narrator sees that every feeling we have is the pain from the crack of the whip and the hurt caused by the lion-tamer's abuse. And these still really hurt. The narrator does not change that hurt; they simply describe its reality in ongoing detail. The narrator also sees all of the ways in which the lion does the bidding for the lion-tamer and describes all of these behaviors in detail. The narrator does not change that behavior; they simply describe its reality in ongoing detail. And in the act of describing both sides of this horrible situation, the narrator starts to see that no matter how loudly the lion-tamer shouts, if there is no lion to do the bidding, then the lion-tamer has no power. In other words, the lion-tamer won't harm you as long as you don't behave like the lion. It doesn't mean their demands or insults will go away; it just means that you don't have to listen to them anymore. For me, this is one of ACT's most striking and fundamental revelations, but it must occur experientially.

Sitting with the mistakes you have already made. The narrator's shoes do not offer any reduction in psychological content or pain, in part because they give the client a 360-degree view of how much of their lives has been spent as the lion and how that played a key role in the current unworkable outcomes. This is a painful place to sit experientially, and the full force of these mistakes can often hit clients very hard. On balance, dealing with this reality provides the perfect opportunity for a first new step for the client, to either wrestle against this fact or to acknowledge and respect it. In ACT, we even go as far as asking clients if they can get comfortable with or even embrace this fact if it will help them to change their behavior. This is what is meant in ACT by the phrase "creative hopelessness," where hopelessness lies in being the lion who performs and creative lies in *seeing* just how much you have been a lion to this point.

Case Erik: part 2

When Erik started therapy, we did not do a standard intake. He had no insight into what causes the tension he experiences when we begin sessions. I've started by asking Erik to tell me what seems relevant to him, and I explore this material further with him while asking more questions to understand why he is where he is. All the time, I keep in mind that it is important that while my knowledge grows, Erik also should gradually gain insight into the story that is playing him now without him realizing it. In the first conversation, Erik mainly talks about himself. During the conversation, it emerges that he sees himself as loyal, flexible, and responsible. He feels that his work does not inspire him enough. He used to have a higher position where he had to constantly meet high demands. He is the only one in his position in his current job. He no longer has to lead a team. At first, he says that this gives him more freedom. He does need input from other teams, and he experiences resistance there. This is one of the reasons why Erik cannot fulfill his assignment. He feels alone in his tasks and responsibilities because he does not receive enough input and support from the other teams. However, he continues to look for the cause and solution of the problem within himself.

I did not take Erik's request for help, "being able to relax more," as a guideline for our interaction. My starting point is that both Erik and I can only know what he really needs if we get to know him better. So I mainly ask questions about how he sees himself in this situation. I want to know what it's like to be Erik and to be so stuck. He only starts to see how trapped he is when I share my observation that he seemed to be trying to meet high standards in his previous position, and he seems to try to meet impossible requirements in his current job. Only then does the insight arise that he is dependent on others to carry out his tasks. He can only now see that it is difficult to relax when there is a lack of cooperation from the other teams. This insight gives Erik access to another piece of his experience that he hadn't been able to see properly before. He realizes that he is becoming even more self-critical in high-demand situations. He can now see that he has continued to blame himself when he was unable to carry out his current assignment properly. Similarly, in subsequent sessions, we continued to explore Erik's self-as-content until all the pieces of the puzzle fell into place.

Summary and conclusions

Clients often enter therapy with a specific, rigid expectation of what change in their lives will look like and will involve in terms of their own behavior. A key aim of ACT is to convert this initial view into a more open, curious exploration of what is workable in this regard. Part of this shift involves helping clients to recognize the unworkability of short-term or painless solutions. Understanding and loosening the grip of self-as-content is the main focus of the current chapter. This involves four key steps. (1) Unpacking the content pieces of the client's story. (2) Seeing how self-as-content pieces work together. (3) Recognizing the client's role in self-as-content. (4) Stepping outside of self-as-content. In all parts of the ACT work here, the therapist's own efforts at personal experiential work provide a useful guide to what the client is being asked to do.

Metaphors, such as McDonald's metaphor, help to direct a client's attention initially to the various pieces of self-as-content, rather than seeing this content in whole cloth. This metaphor also presents the idea that some of these pieces are perceived as positive, while others are perceived as negative. In a nutshell, clients are juggling with a sense of stuckness between these two types of self-as-content. The Ham Sandwich Metaphor is helpful in enabling clients to touch this painful sense of stuckness. However, what clients initially present with is typically negative, painful content that dominates their attention, such as anxiety or pain. In spite of this dominance, it is important that therapy here is slow in order to let this content emerge without making any efforts to change it. Although this might feel pointless or too slow, something very useful is happening, as the client is learning to observe and talk about that content from the perspective of another human being.

There is a delicate balance to be struck here between recognizing the extent to which the client feels helpless and the fact that their own behavior is part of what keeps things the way they are. The way these two opposing forces are reconciled is to present it to the client that it is understandable that they simply cannot help doing what they are doing while things remain as they are. The key message is to fully appreciate the almost compulsive, can't-help-it way in which your actions follow your mind's instructions. The lion-tamer metaphor is particularly useful in this regard and for facilitating future therapeutic directions. The fact that the same behavior will always produce the same outcome is an important experiential insight for clients here.

Taking up the position of narrator is a useful metaphor for stepping outside of self-as-content. However, it is critical for the client to fully appreciate that this new perspective will not reduce ongoing pain. The narrator does not change that hurt; they simply describe its reality in ongoing detail. Indeed, the narrator's perspective begins to see the mistakes that have already been made, and as a result, pain or distress might actually increase. This is a key distinction in ACT that takes a long time to really wrestle with. In ACT, we even go as far as asking clients if they can get comfortable or even embrace this increased pain if it will help them to change their behavior. This is what is meant in ACT by the phrase "creative hopelessness." Understanding the pieces of self-as-content and directing our therapeutic efforts to enable clients to step outside of this content allows them to break out of the hopelessness of previous unworkable change efforts and move toward a more creative position in which workable change can begin to be facilitated.

Reference

Hayes, S. C., & McCurry, S. M. (1989). *Comprehensive distancing. A manual for the treatment of emotional avoidance*. Department of Psychology, University of Nevada.

Chapter 3

Understanding and weakening fusion through defusion interventions

Ciara McEnteggart and Yvonne Barnes-Holmes

This chapter aims to introduce you to the acceptance and commitment therapy (ACT) concepts of fusion and defusion so that you can learn to design defusion-based interventions that will essentially free your clients from the demands and pressures of their internal experiences. We will emphasize throughout how fully appreciating fusion and defusion will enable you to create the most precise and targeted defusion techniques for each of your clients.

We have divided defusion interventions into five areas, which you can follow as a rough sequence, but we also urge serious caution not to embrace defusion in a strictly stage-like way. The key components of defusion we discuss are: using analogy and metaphor; weakening the literal meaning of internal experiences; distinguishing self from these experiences; distancing these experiences from self; and weakening the behavioral control of these experiences in the client's life.

At the beginning and end of the chapter, we summarize a client with whom defusion interventions proved highly effective but where they were not straightforward. The chapter contains other real-life client examples. We have also presented personal exercises for you to engage in, in order for you to fully experience the power of fusion and defusion with regard to your own internal experiences and the aspects of your behavior directed by these.

Introduction to defusion

There has been much written about defusion and its counterpart of cognitive distancing. Both can be viewed as interventions that are designed to distance the client from some aspect of their internal experience which causes distress and has unwanted control over their behavior. But if you *fully* appreciate the parallel concepts of fusion and defusion, you can design defusion interventions in ACT that do much more than distancing.

Case analysis Emily: part 1

To open the chapter in a clinically meaningful way, we have summarized below the context of a client with whom defusion interventions were a critical feature of her

DOI: 10.4324/9781032699691-4

engagement with us in ACT. Toward the end of the chapter, we revisit this client and summarize the defusion-based techniques we used to help her overcome this painful problem with fusion.

Emily was a lady in her mid-60s who had been diagnosed in the previous year with stomach cancer. The diagnosis had taken her completely by surprise because she had been largely asymptomatic and the cancer was inadvertently discovered during an alternative routine medical checkup. After surgery and a short bout of drug treatment, her prognosis appeared good, and she remained cancer-free at the time of her referral for psychological help.

She was advised to undertake individual therapy because she was unwilling to attend group sessions for patients with similar medical issues. Specifically, she argued that she "did not want to be dragged down by other patients' negativity." The medical professional recognized a similar pattern of behavior around her family, where she felt fear and shame about being a further burden on them. Paradoxically, concealing her worries was interfering with her ability to closely connect with her family at this difficult time.

A recent example of this occurred on holiday, where she and her husband were out walking, and she began thinking about him walking alone after she dies. As she got wrapped up in these painful images, she felt the closeness with her husband slip away, and this convinced her even more that she was a burden to him and should stop sharing her worries.

From an ACT perspective, one can certainly say that Emily was fused with these ongoing health worries and the sense that they made her a burden to her family. Indeed, these fears had excessive, unwanted control over important aspects of her behavior around them.

What is fusion?

We could not fully discuss the concept of defusion or illustrate defusion-based interventions without first exploring the parallel concept of fusion. According to the 1.5.5 Learner's (English) Dictionary, the term fusion means "the process or result of joining two or more things together to form one." In line with this definition, the way fusion is used in ACT describes the joining of a client's sense of self with some aspect of that person's internal experience. Consider the simple example of a client who recurrently has thoughts about being a bad person and soon begins to believe they really are a bad person. In this case, fusion describes the belief that the presence of the thoughts *makes* them a bad person (i.e., 'I am what I think'). As a result of this joining of the person (self) with the thoughts (being bad), painful feelings that accompany these thoughts also become part of the fusion, and eventually the negative thoughts and feelings gain increasing amounts of control over behavior, especially through emotional avoidance.

Let's do a simple personal exercise using the text box below. Think about the worst possible criticism anyone could ever have of you, even if it never happened. We want you to think of something bad that someone might say about you that would really hurt. Then we want you to write it in the box below as a statement about you. For example, your worst possible criticism might be: "I am a very self-ish person." So, begin the statement with the words "I am..."

Fusion exercise

Please write your answer here.
I am...

Notice, just how painful that statement is when you read it. And part of that pain comes from some (even small) element of believability, where the statement might just have a grain of truth and thus it might say something fundamental about the type of person you think you are. That is fusion because it joins the statement about you with you as a real person.

From an ACT perspective, the presence of negative thoughts and feelings in and of themselves is not problematic, but difficulties arise for all of us when these experiences are believed to be *true* indicators of the self (i.e., when *fusion* occurs). The actions that then accompany these internal experiences are further appraised as evidence of reality, thus strengthening the thoughts and feelings and deepening the fusion. The more actions these internal experiences take hold of, the more the person will identify with this behavior (e.g., 'I am what I do') and with the internal experiences that direct it ('I am what I think and feel'). This fusion naturally encourages emotional avoidance, in part because of the deep distress it encompasses (e.g., 'I can't manage my children, therefore I must be a terrible mother').

Where does fusion come from?

For ACT, fusion is a natural by-product of complex human language abilities, and its development is largely unavoidable. The high prevalence in the general population of psychological suffering that requires help certainly supports this account. However, the presence of negative or painful thoughts and feelings does not *necessarily* predict the fusion of these with one's identity. The trouble begins when negative thoughts about the self combine with painful feelings, and this com-bination gains power typically through unwillingness to talk about or share these experiences, and thus emotional avoidance sets in. Acceptance (often implicit in sharing with others) is a powerful prophylactic against fusion because when we approach and accept our thoughts and feelings, they are less likely to control what we do. It is in this way that ACT's components of defusion and acceptance are closely bound together.

Fusion and behavioral control

One of the key reasons why clients come to therapy is the fact that they repeatedly engage in actions that have negative consequences, but which they perceive they cannot control. In other words, much of their behavior is *not* based on choices or values, but rather on fusion and avoidance. In this respect, ACT's concept of fusion is similar to the term 'thought-action fusion' (Shafran et al., 1996) first proposed to understand clinical obsessions. What both concepts see as problematic for clients is the incorrect assumption that *in and of themselves thoughts can and even must* directly influence external events, such as behavior.

Again, let's do a personal exercise. Think about two actions you do regularly and which you try hard to stop but can't. This could include something large, like trying to quit smoking or over-eating, or it could be smaller, like trying to stop using swear words. Whatever it is, let it be something that you've tried hard to stop doing, but it never seems to happen, and part of you just doesn't fully understand why you can't change. Where behavioral change on the surface seems simple, but you repeatedly fail to do it, is a typical place where fusion exists.

> ### Fusion and behavioral control exercise
>
> **Please write your answers here.**
> Example. I am too critical of others and I'd really like to stop.
> 1.
> 2.

In the short exercise above, we could have asked you to write a list of ten things you do that are based on fusion, but we didn't do that simply because you wouldn't have been able to see them clearly. Indeed, one feature of fusion is that because the meanings of self that it contains are so well established, all of the actions you do at one level feel as if you are choosing to do them. Yet, at another level, the opposite appears to be the case, and that is why it is so hard for you to change that behavior.

In your clinical work, we want you to recognize that no-one is fully or correctly aware of all aspects of the behavioral control that their fusion has acquired. So, even if you ask clients repeatedly about this, they won't be able to answer fully or correctly. Nonetheless, as a clinician, you need to fully appreciate the extent of behavioral control that fusion can acquire, and we often work with ACT clinicians who underestimate this. Specifically, they sometimes target individual negative thoughts (e.g., catastrophizing about illness) and the actions they produce (avoiding the doctor), while failing to see the full picture of behavioral control fusion has over a client's life. The ACT concept of fusion, therefore, places erosion of the sense of self at its core, and it is based on this that we expect that a great deal of behavior is under the control of fusion.

The example below of one of our clients illustrates the extent of behavioral control that fusion can acquire and the damage this can quickly cause. Notice, as you read, how quickly the client's struggle evolves in the space of a day and how random contextual variables can easily become part of the struggle. Notice how her sense of self-worth is easily drawn into the situation.

Client example of fusion and behavioral control

A married woman with children does not work outside of the home. One day, she experiences rushing thoughts while doing the grocery shopping (e.g., 'I don't see why I have to do all the menial family tasks like shopping. I could do more with my life than this'). Even though she had these thoughts before, they now feel particularly salient (because she had tense words with her husband the night before).

When the woman returns home from shopping, she is increasingly troubled by these thoughts and starts to feel frustration and tension across her chest. As she thinks through where the thoughts are coming from, she pieces together: the tense words with her husband; the fact that he has on several occasions been away with friends without her; and his recent stress at work, which has meant that they have had little time together. As these recollections coincide, her frustration increases and new thoughts occur, such as 'Perhaps my husband is having an affair' and 'Maybe I don't love him anymore'. Naturally, these new worries appear more serious, and she feels even more tense. The thought that she may no longer love him sits particularly heavily at the front of her mind.

That evening when her husband comes home, she is distant and awkward with him as she starts to feel confused about their relationship and guilty about her recent doubts. Stressed out from another day at work, he reacts negatively to her coldness and is derogatory about the fact that she did not have to "work" that day, while he did. After this exchange, she is hurt and more convinced that she no longer loves him, with the emergence of new thoughts, such as 'Someone who loved me would not think I was so useless'.

This example illustrates what we call the 'domino effect' of fusion involving thoughts, feelings, actions, and the self. While some aspects of the client's situation above may have even been random or irrelevant, they exerted a direct negative influence on the interactions between the couple, which may well have done their relationship lasting damage.

How to detect fusion in therapy

You cannot see or measure fusion directly; it is not a behavioral process. It is simply a useful way, as ACT clinicians, to describe how aspects of the client's experience (e.g., thoughts and feelings) encroach upon their sense of self or identity and acquire unwanted control over their behavior. Hence, you should be assessing fusion early on by looking for examples of *which* thoughts and feelings hold the most powerful meanings for a client's sense of self, and which client actions these meanings appear to control. Consider the brief description given by a client below. Notice how genuinely the client sounds like they are making a valued choice.

Example for detecting fusion early in therapy

No-one understands what it feels like to be so anxious. It's just not possible for me to go to the shops when the panic strikes. I can't do that to myself. It's better for me to stay at home. That is really all I want to do.

This example already says a lot about the client in terms of fusion. First, it shows how limited the client's action-based choices have become when the feelings are intense. That is, the client sees no workable alternative to doing exactly what the anxious thoughts and feelings dictate. Second, and more subtly, you can get a sense of how much bigger the feelings are than the client. In simple terms, part of their identity appears to have been taken over by these experiences and the need to act upon them. Again, this example suggests that your clinical work should not stop at individual thoughts and feelings, but you should remain aware of the whole picture of behavioral functions that fusion can acquire.

What is defusion?

In simple terms, defusion is the opposite of fusion and describes a situation in which an individual's internal experiences are perceived as separate from their identity, and as such, they exert only limited control over behavior. However, it is important that you do not to see defusion as a state or behavioral style; rather, it is best for you to see it as a current behavioral repertoire that does not contain fusion and where actions are driven by personal choices, rather than by fusion and avoidance.

We typically reserve the term defusion for descriptions of the ACT-based interventions we use to tackle fusion, and our understanding of the concept of fusion directs the focus of these techniques. In short, your defusion interventions should lead to the weakening of fusion by separating the client's identity from specific internal experiences and reducing the extent to which these influence behavior. Where this separation of self from experience has not occurred, we would say that your defusion interventions have not worked or have not been undertaken fully. In the sections below, we explore examples of where defusion-based interventions, in our experience, cannot weaken or break fusion.

What defusion interventions involve

Weakening fusion as a therapeutic aim is far from easy because by the time clients enter therapy, thoughts and feelings have already taken hold of many aspects of their daily behavioral repertoires. Indeed, this is why defusion interventions feature at the beginning of ACT's treatment regime. In the sections below, we will outline the critical features of defusion, including: using analogy and metaphor in defusion interventions; weakening the literal meaning of internal experiences; distinguishing self from these experiences; distancing these experiences from self; and weakening the behavioral control of these experiences in the client's life.

The role of analogy and metaphor in defusion interventions

Prior to delving into defusion interventions, we want to draw your attention to the large extent to which analogy and metaphor figure in these techniques. Of course, analogy and metaphor have a long-established history as therapeutic tools in perhaps most psychotherapy regimes. Indeed, they facilitate two vital achievements. First, they validate the client's experience. Second, they enhance the client's awareness of their own situation, with a view to opening up new solutions. However, two additional and related features of the use of analogy and metaphor distinguish ACT from practically all other treatment regimes. The first of these is the sheer extent to which ACT clinicians use these linguistic tools, which generally exceeds what therapists do in other treatment programs. The second feature accounts for this reliance because the use of analogy and metaphor is one of the most powerful aspects of defusion interventions that enable them to weaken fusion. We explain this below using the early ACT concept of deliteralization.

In the early days of ACT, the concept of deliteralization was used to describe the weakening of what is now known as fusion and particularly the reduction of its behavioral control in a client's life (Hayes et al., 1999). 'Deliteralization' specifically referred to reducing the literal functions or believability of internal experiences, so that they no longer appeared to define the self or signify one's identity. In other words, the literal meaning or function of internal experiences (fusion) was being reduced. For example, if a client regularly has the thought "I'm depressed," that often means (literally) for that client that they are a depressed person. In other words, rather than the client seeing this experience as a thought they have, it functions literally to tell them who they are. You can easily see how the concept of literal functions became the concept of fusion because they are based on the same core idea of internal experiences joining with the sense of self.

Analogy and metaphor are non-literal linguistic structures that often coordinate stimuli that are not typically coordinated in everyday language. For example, you might describe your child as a puppy, because they are cute and playful, even though in literal language, puppies and children are very different. Indeed, analogy and metaphor offer a metaphorical view (like story-telling) that differs from a literal view (e.g., children are not the same as puppies). What is happening here is a shift from a literal view of those stimuli to a looser, metaphorical view of those stimuli, thus altering one's perception of them. Similarly, when analogy and metaphor are used in therapy, they shift the client's relationship with their own experiences from a literal view (I am what I think and feel) to a *metaphorical* view. Consider the therapeutic analogy below, which we frequently use with clients.

The anxiety as a river analogy

I can see how those anxious feelings just sweep you away like a strong river. Then the river tosses you up ragged on the shore when it is done with you.

This metaphor of the feelings as a river shifts the client's literal view of 'I am anxious' to a more metaphorical view of 'my anxiety is like a river that can overcome me and leave me exhausted'. This shift in the client's perspective on their own anxiety is a core feature of defusion. Hence, your defusion interventions *should* comprise a great deal of analogy and metaphor, and in ACT, this is typically the case.

Let's try to be creative and use analogy or metaphor to deliteralize a strong personal feeling with which you might experience fusion. In the box below, identify one powerful feeling you get regularly which makes you very uncomfortable and which you try to avoid. Then try to construct a simple metaphor that captures what that feeling does to you when it shows up, similar to the river metaphor above for feeling anxious.

Creating a metaphor for fusion exercise

Please write your answers here.
Write the feeling you try to avoid here...
Below, create a metaphor that describes what that feeling does to you when it occurs.

Of course, there are many other ways we can experience a shift in our perspective of our own internal experiences, such as through direct experience, instructions, rules, etc. But, when used in therapy, analogy and metaphor offer a non-threatening and effective means of achieving this shift and ultimately facilitating defusion. In our experience, analogy and metaphor are the least intrusive and most effective means of shifting perspective in this way. As you will see in the sections that follow, many defusion exercises involve metaphorical shifts in one's perspective of their own experience.

Weakening the literal meaning of internal experiences

Based on the original concept of deliteralization, early versions of ACT relied heavily on word repetition exercises to begin defusion. In simple terms, repeating a word over and over reduces its literal meaning, as the word becomes just a sound. Indeed, word repetition exercises are aimed at what is called 'semantic satiation' (e.g., Espositio & Phelton, 1971). Read the exercise below, then try to do it yourself and notice how meaning changes profoundly in a short time.

The milk milk milk word repetition exercise (Titchener, 1916)

Let's take a simple random word that you're very familiar with. Let's select the word "milk." Before we do anything with this word, let's explore what it really means to you right now, in terms of what you understand about it. What shows up as you think about that word in your mind? Probably you're thinking of its creamy color and light texture. Perhaps you prefer to drink it cold. Maybe you can imagine the taste of it and think about whether or not you like that taste. So, now we can see that the word "milk" has quite a few meanings for you attached to it.

Now, let's see what happens when we try to change those meanings with a silly game. Please say the word "milk" out loud. Now say it again. And again. And again. Now start saying it over and over, and don't stop. And as you're doing that, begin to say it louder and louder. And as you are getting louder, start to also speed up, so that you're saying the word faster and faster. Do this until you just can't say the word "milk" anymore.

Now, let's think about what just happened to the word "milk." First, it started off in the usual way with you thinking the things about it that you have always thought. But then something happened, and that stuff disappeared. And as it disappeared, something new appeared in its place. Probably that was a squeaky, strange sound that the original word just collapsed into, and it almost became something you didn't even recognize.

In this exercise, the properties that have been established for you of the stimulus "milk" slipped away, and the word lost its literal meaning, at least temporarily. This is precisely what we want to do with clients with the words or stimuli that participate in fusion, but we make it non-intrusive to begin with by using a simple neutral word, such as "milk." With clients, we then repeat the exercise with more clinically relevant words and phrases (e.g., 'I'm depressed') in order to establish the same effect, but now an internal experience is the target.

The next exercise asks you to do just that. Try to think of something negative or judgmental about yourself that often shows up in your mind. Don't be tempted to think of something trivial. Instead, try to select something that bothers you a lot and that you wish you didn't have. This might be a self-judgment like "I'm stupid" or "I made a mistake." Or it could be a rhetorical question that you always ask yourself, such as "Why can't I change?"

Word repetition exercise for a recurrent negative thought about you

Please write your thought here.

Now, let's explore what that thought really means to you when it pops into your mind. Bring it into your mind right now slowly. What comes up as you think about it? Probably you're starting to feel something. Now, you can really see what that thought really means to you, and it probably means a lot more than you realized before.

Now, let's see what happens when we play the same silly game with your thought, as we just played with "milk." Please say your thought out loud. Now say it again. And again. And again. Now start saying it over and over, and don't stop. And as you're doing that, begin to say it louder and louder. And now, as you are getting louder, start to also speed up, so that you're saying the words faster and faster. Do this until you just can't say that sentence anymore.

Now, let's look at what is left of what that thought used to mean to you. It probably doesn't make you feel anything anymore. It probably doesn't connect to anything it used to connect to. It probably just feels like nonsense. The point here is this. If what that thought means really matters, how come that all just slips away so quickly?

This loosening of meaning is an essential first step in weakening fusion because it helps clients to begin to see that thoughts are just collections of words and not reflections of reality or the self. However, several caveats seem important here. First, the reduction in literal meanings is often temporary, and they may quickly return to the client's natural environment. Second, breaking literal meaning should not come across as the therapist invalidating what a client thinks or believes. Third, these exercises should not have any hint that the distress associated with the thought will be reduced as a result of the repetition (because this would only serve to enhance the thought's existing avoidant functions).

Distinguishing self from internal experiences

Referring collectively to "The Mind" as the keeper of all internal experiences is one of ACT's most established metaphors and is typically employed at the beginning of defusion interventions, after the word repetition exercises above. The core aim of this metaphor is to begin the separation of the self from internal experiences by simply *distinguishing* the two from each other and collectively referring to these experiences as the content of the Mind. It is important to note that because the stimulus Mind usually refers to something internal, there is no attempt here to distance the client from the Mind in terms of placing the Mind outside oneself. That would likely be difficult for a client who is very fused with their internal experiences. As such, the Mind metaphor simply collects all internal experiences together and distinguishes them from the person having them, but it is not yet driving at any form of distancing, which at this very early stage in therapy would likely be a step too far. Nonetheless, you can already see how established literal meaning would begin to loosen (i.e., I am not my Mind's experiences).

There are many aspects of the Mind metaphor that we use in early defusion interventions to repeatedly strengthen this distinction between self and Mind's internal experiences. The box below includes some of the ones we use most often.

The mind metaphor: strengthening distinction between self and experience

1. We ask clients, "What is your Mind saying to you right now?"
2. We ask clients to get into the habit of saying: "I'm having the thought that…"
3. We ask clients to say: "Thank-you, Mind, for giving me that thought."
4. We ask clients to say a thought aloud, and then, with the client, we sing that thought like a song.
5. We ask clients to say a thought aloud, and then we repeat the thought back in a silly voice.

Another powerful tool we use for distinguishing Mind from self when the above has been successful is what we refer to as the Four People Scenario, which we present to clients as follows.

Metaphor: the four people scenario

It seems that there are actually four of us in this room, and not just two. There is you and your Mind, and there is me and my Mind. That makes four, not two. And when there are four personalities in the room, things get much busier and noisier because now there are four characters competing for attention and space, rather than just two who can take turns. What seems to happen when all four of us get in here and we all start talking over one another is that your Mind starts to dominate and really wants to be heard. Then you, and sometimes even I, feel like we have to just sit quietly and be forced to hear what your Mind insists on telling us. That can feel very disempowering, even for me, and I'm sure especially for you.

In order to enhance the experiential aspect of the Mind metaphor and to clearly show how internal experiences dominate, ACT clinicians typically extend the metaphor into a physical exercise called Taking Your Mind for a Walk. The first part is below. The core aim of the exercise at this point is to highlight the sheer volume of internal experiences the client has, which is easier to see when they are spoken aloud as soon as they emerge. This exercise is from Hayes et al. (1999).

Taking your mind for a walk exercise: part 1

In this physical exercise, we are going to ask you to get up from your chair and walk around the room for several minutes. As you are walking, we want you to begin to say aloud all of the thoughts your Mind generates on an ongoing basis. Just say every single thing that pops into your Mind, the instant it pops in.

Pay particular attention to what your Mind says about what you're actually doing here. It will probably tell you, "You look stupid." Say all that stuff out loud too.

In the next part of the exercise, we add an instruction that asks the client not to do what the Mind suggests. For example, if the thought 'I should stop this and sit down' pops up, we ask the client to keep walking and not do what the thought suggests.

Taking your mind for a walk exercise: part 2

In this next part of the exercise, we want you to repeat the exercise again, but this time we want you to pay particular attention when your Mind gives you any instructions or directions on what you should do. For example, your Mind might tell you to sit down with the thought, "You look ridiculous, you should just sit down." When Mind gives you any instructions on what to do, we want you to explicitly ignore that instruction and just keep walking around the room, saying your thoughts aloud.

It is clear how this aspect of the exercise is designed to tackle the literal functions of the thoughts because the client is explicitly instructed not to do what any thought says. Although we are still at the distinguishing self from experience stage of defusion, we are already beginning to reduce the behavioral control of internal experiences. This aspect of the exercise often resonates with clients who feel that they have no genuine control over much of their behavior, and the possibility of a different type of control or choice slowly begins to emerge.

Before moving on to the next section, we would strongly encourage you to now do both parts of the Taking Your Mind for a Walk Exercise. As you do, notice any recurrent thoughts your Mind gives you. Check what form these most often take. Perhaps they are judgments, statements, or instructions. Notice also what shows up when you explicitly refuse to do what your Mind suggests.

Distancing internal experiences from self

Once the distinguishing between the client and their Mind has been established, defusion interventions shift notably toward distancing self from Mind and thus from the internal experiences it generates. The aim of distancing, of course, is again to create separation from the self, but the focus now is to view internal experiences from an external perspective, thus changing the existing perspective the client has on their internal world. This is what was meant by the original ACT term, 'comprehensive distancing'. In simple terms, clients now see these experiences as *outside* of themselves, rather than seeing them as *inside* (i.e., placing them out there instead of in here). Once again, it is important to remind you that you should never imply in your distancing techniques with clients that a reduction in distress will be achieved, lest avoidance functions get inadvertently strengthened. You have probably already witnessed instances of clients distancing from painful thoughts or self-judgments in order to avoid them. Even though this is distancing, its avoidant function means it cannot be part of a defusion strategy.

One of our favorite ACT physical exercises for beginning distancing in defusion, called The Hands over Eyes Exercise, is presented below. This is a simple physical exercise that offers the perfect analog to the psychological distancing we are trying to achieve in defusion techniques. Once you have read and familiarized yourself with the exercise, we would ask you to physically do the exercise for yourself and see what you notice afterwards.

The hands over eyes exercise

Place both hands over your face and keep your fingers all close together. Now open your eyes underneath your hands. All you can see from that place is your hands. They look large, dark, and red, and they stop you seeing anything else, even though it might be close by.

Now, just pull your hands a few inches from your face and look at your fingers once again. Now you see them and everything else differently. Your fingers are bright and skin-colored, and you can see other things around them.

Starting to look at the thoughts and feelings we have inside is a bit like this. When they are inside, they look dark and large, and they stop us from seeing anything around them. But when we imagine them in front of us, like writing them down on a piece of paper, they begin to look very different, and you can see that they too have stuff around them.

So, just like taking your hands away from your face, I'm asking you to place your thoughts and feelings on the table in front of you, so that we don't get that distorted view of them that we get when they are inside you.

The physicality of distancing in this exercise will be obvious to you, but it is also important to note that the exercise highlights a key benefit of distancing in terms of clarifying the reality of what one is seeing (i.e., a thought is just a thought). This highlights for the client that their existing internal view is likely to be skewed or distorted. When you actually did the exercise for yourself, can you fully contact how distorted the world looks when your hands are too close up to your face?

Pointing out this distortion in the perspective on their internal world with which clients enter therapy is an important aspect of defusion that comes through in our work on distancing. At a technical level, what we are trying to do here is to reduce the appetitive and literal meaning of internal experiences and make them more aversive. In simple language, the client learns that seeing experiences from an internal perspective is distorted and cannot be trusted. One metaphor we use at this point with almost all clients really emphasizes this view of an internal, distorted reality. The Kaleidoscope Glasses metaphor is presented below. The more the client learns to distrust their mind, the more likely it is that the therapist will be able to distance the client from Mind's experiences.

The Kaleidoscope glasses metaphor

Your Mind seems to have a very distinct way of looking at things. It's like you walk around wearing a pair of those kaleidoscope glasses that make the world look distorted and make you dizzy. It seems like everything you see is from that distorted lens. Nothing looks real or clear; everything looks wobbly, and you can't be sure of it. Even your thoughts, feelings, and sensations seem to get distorted with those glasses on, and it's scary because you don't know what to believe or trust.

Let's again do a simple personal exercise. Try to think clearly about three distortions your Mind makes about you, which you don't always see as a distortion. For example, your Mind might regularly call you "stupid" even though you do many clever things. In the box below, we want you to write a list of three key distortions your Mind does, as well as the reasons why you think each is a distortion. For example, Mind says, "you get everything wrong," and yet you know that you don't get everything wrong, only some things. Consider again that because of fusion, there are probably many distortions your Mind is making and which you never see at all.

Exercise distortions from your Kaleidoscope glasses

Distortion 1
  Mind says:
  Reality is:

Distortion 2
  Mind says:
  Reality is:

Distortion 3
  Mind says:
  Reality is:

Physicality, such as in the Hands over Eyes Exercise, is a common theme in distancing work, which uses physical metaphors to help the client experience *physical* distance from their internal experiences. This theme is also evident in an extension to the Taking Your Mind for a Walk Exercise that has been in ACT since the beginning; see below. What the addition of the therapist as the client's Mind serves to do here is to enhance the physical distance between the client and their internal experiences, because these are not only now made external, but they are even being reported by a different person.

Exercise taking your mind for a walk: part 3

After presenting the first part of this exercise as described above, we then bring the therapist into the exercise by having both the client and the therapist walk around the room together. Typically, the therapist now walks behind the client and pretends to be the client's Mind thinking aloud. As the therapist says aloud all the thoughts that are most likely to show up for the client, the client is again instructed to simply listen to the Mind, while continuing to do the exercise (e.g., continue walking around the room, even if the Mind tells you to sit down).

It would simply feel remiss of us at this point if we did not mention the famous Leaves on the Stream Exercise (Hayes, 2005), which has been used by ACT clinicians for so long in defusion interventions that are focused on distancing.

The leaves on the stream exercise: part 1

Clients are simply instructed to imagine themselves sitting on the bank at the edge of a stream. As each thought emerges in real time, the client is asked to: note the thought; place it on a leaf; place that leaf on the stream; and watch it slip away.

Again, the physical distancing in this metaphor is obvious, and the stream can be long, thus enhancing distance even further. In addition, we have found that emphasizing a piece at the end of the metaphor helps alert clients to see how easy it is to 'fall into the stream' with thoughts that are particularly sticky (i.e., the ones that have the strongest behavioral functions).

The leaves on the stream exercise: part 2

As part of the exercise, clients are asked to be aware that some thoughts that are hard to place on a leaf will actually pull them off the bank, and before they realize it, they're in the stream getting wet, still holding onto that leaf. When this happens, clients are asked to lift the leaf back out of the water, along with themselves, re-position themselves back safely up on the bank further away from the water. And, when they're ready, try again with that leaf, making sure this time that they let it go quickly in order to avoid getting pulled in again.

Before moving on to the next section, we would strongly encourage you to now do the Leaves on the Stream Exercise for yourself, making sure that you consider both parts. To do the exercise fully, it takes around 20 minutes.

When clients are not ready for distancing

It makes sense that further separation of self from experience cannot be tackled if at least some level of distance has not been established. Nonetheless, it is important to emphasize that distancing is often harder to achieve than it might first seem (because of fusion), and the path to distancing itself is fraught with obstacles. Indeed, we have struggled to achieve distance with many clients, especially where they see their internal experiences as hugely valuable or salient (e.g., with chronic pain or unusual experiences). We provide an example below of this type of client with whom we have experienced real obstacles to our attempts to create distance, and we also illustrate how we overcame those obstacles.

Client example of difficulty in distancing

We once saw a middle-aged woman who had experienced chronic pain for many years and could no longer work as a result. It was relatively easy to distinguish this client from her experiences of pain and the thoughts and feelings that surrounded it, because she saw all of these as negative things she really did not want to have in her life.

We then attempted to distance the client from these experiences to highlight that they were all part of a real, valid bigger picture of pain that had now become a huge part of her life.

But we simply could not get this client to see this larger picture as outside of herself and as something that now dominated her every action. Indeed, although we had worked hard to validate the client's pain and related experiences, it seemed as if our attempts to distance her from them diminished her suffering in some way. Naturally, she resisted this because these experiences had become such a big part of her identity (fusion).

What was distinctive about this and similar clients is the extent to which their identity has become largely defined by their pain, disability, or illness. Indeed, this also figures strongly in their family relationships (e.g., 'my mum is sick all the time'). In short, we might say that fusion is particularly strong here, as the client has now come to identify with her 'sick role'. In order to avoid invalidating this identity, it is important to keep the experiences located internally and to highlight the large amount of space they take up. Indeed, we fully appreciated that she felt that she had no choice but to let her experiences and actions be dominated by this identity. The box below describes what we did next with this client instead of distancing.

Resolution for client example of difficulty in distancing

In the next intervention with this client, we acknowledged that her suffering was huge and that she had no choice but to try to ameliorate it in whatever way she could.

Specifically, we proposed that pain was large but she was small, and no matter how hard she tried to deal with it or help herself, the pain situation just seemed to get worse and worse.

We then introduced a metaphor to validate the fact that the pain was large and that she was small in comparison and thus had no control over the pain itself. The metaphor we employed here is called Master and Servant, and we use it with a lot of clients at this point.

Pain is the master, and the client is the servant who has been loyal and practical. But serving this master leaves no time, space, or energy for serving any other master, such as herself, her relationships with loved ones, or even her job. The pain master is relentless, and no matter how hard you work for them, it's never enough. So, you just become more and more trapped and enslaved, while the master seems to grow stronger and stronger as a result of your hard work.

The Master and Servant metaphor validates the dominance of pain without evaluating it negatively. Rather, it simply acknowledges how demanding pain is and how it is never satisfied. It is important to note that this is more than distinguishing self from experience, but it does not go as far as distancing. In simple terms, the shift in perspective we are pushing here is one of big (pain)-small (client), rather than inside–outside that is typically the object of distancing and which some clients experience as diminishing and invalidating.

Weakening the behavioral control of internal experiences

When the distinguishing and distancing aspects of defusion have been established, there is still work to do on reducing the behavioral functions that have become attached to internal experiences. Let us be explicit, distinguishing and distancing in and of themselves will often not adequately reduce the behavioral functions that fusion has acquired.

In the sections above, we have already seen examples of early defusion interventions that begin to weaken the behavioral functions of fusion. Remember the Four People Scenario and how the client's Mind can make the client and the therapist say less. Remember the instruction for clients during the Taking Your Mind for a Walk Exercise to keep walking. Recall how acknowledging the distortion in the Hands over Eyes Exercise and in the Kaleidoscope Glasses metaphor suggests that clients should not do what thoughts say because they give a distorted view of reality. Also, recall the Leaves on the Stream Exercise and the piece at the end that instructs clients to return to the bank and stay out of the water.

ACT has many additional ways of reducing the behavioral functions of fusion that build on the distinguishing and distancing pieces above, and which remain central to our defusion interventions. These may be subtle, such as using the verb "buying" to refer to doing what your thoughts tell you. "Buying" is a very active verb and encourages clients to see themselves following the thoughts' instructions as active rather than passive. In a simple analogy, thoughts are also described as bullies who force you to do what they want. The Feeding the Tiger metaphor also helps clients to see that there will be negative consequences for following Mind's instructions (Hayes, 2005).

Feeding the tiger metaphor

Suppose you come home from work and there is a tiger cub sitting at your back door. He is still very small, and he whines softly. You take him inside with you, and you give him something to eat to make him stop whining. Then you give him a box with a blanket in it to sleep in. You go to bed and don't think anything about it anymore. The next morning, you hear a soft whining as you come down the stairs, and you think: He's hungry, let's quickly feed the tiger.

And every time you feed the tiger, he grows. And every day, he roars a little louder. And one day, you start feeding him because you're afraid of that tiger, not because he is small and hungry. We often treat the painful pieces of our history the same way.

One key ACT metaphor that is particularly effective at reducing the behavioral functions of fusion is the Passengers on the Bus metaphor (Hayes et al., 1999).

Passengers on the bus metaphor

In this scenario, negative thoughts in particular are described as nasty passengers on a bus that represents the client's life (client is the driver).

The metaphor emphasizes that these passengers are frightening and bully the driver, ultimately to get control over the bus.

The metaphor stresses how at each turn in the road, the bullies want to dictate the direction the bus takes at the cost of the client's own wishes about where they want their life to go.

We often extend this metaphor in order to focus on this latter piece about choices, and we include numerous examples, one after the other, of directions the bullies might want versus the directions that the client would choose. This them-versus-you piece is particularly effective at showing the client the cost of living in accordance with the behavioral functions of fusion. In short, the metaphor highlights that fusion disregards what the client wants, and thus they are disempowered from making their own choices. This explicit distinction not only weakens the functions of fusion but also begins to establish new behavioral functions, especially choosing for yourself. In more general technical terms, one might say that what is happening in this part of defusion interventions is that the functions of fusion, such as doing what thoughts say, are being deactivated (behavioral deactivation), while new functions, such as choosing, are being activated (behavioral activation).

Using the text box below, we would like you to work through the Passengers on the Bus metaphor for yourself. Make a list of the three nastiest passengers (thoughts, feelings, etc.) that are regularly on your bus. Note what each one tries to force you to do. Think about what you might really want to do instead.

Passengers on your bus exercise

Please write your answers here.
List the three nastiest passengers that are regularly on your bus.

Passenger 1:
What does this passenger try to force you to do?

....
....
....
....
....
....

What might YOU want to do instead?

....
....
....
....

Passenger 2:
What does this passenger try to force you to do?

....
....
....

What might YOU want to do instead?

....

....

....

Passenger 3:
What does this passenger try to force you to do?

....

....

....

What might YOU want to do instead?

....

....

....

Separation of self from internal experiences

Throughout the sections above, we have emphasized the centrality of the self in ACT's concept of fusion and in our defusion interventions. We structured the current chapter by dividing our defusion work into four sections that weave through a rough but non-prescribed sequence as follows: weakening the literal meaning of internal experiences; distinguishing self from these experiences; distancing self; and weakening behavioral control by fusion. As noted above, these sections follow that sequence. For example, distancing could not be fully established if there was no distinction between self and experiences. And yet, it should also be clear to you that each stage provides subtle opportunities for you as the clinician to set up what will come next. Specifically, every aspect of defusion work is ultimately about separating the self from one's experience, so this should not be seen as the final step, given that this would not be possible until the pieces before it had been established. It is also important to recognize the caveats that we noted above, where obstacles to defusion are frequently encountered. It is for these reasons that we firmly believe that it is extremely difficult, if not impossible, to protocolize defusion-based work. In this sense, defusion should be tailored to each client's individual situation.

As well as noting the special challenges we have witnessed in our defusion work with clients with chronic pain and disability or those who report unusual experiences, this chapter would be lacking if we did not mention the specific difficulties we have experienced in doing defusion interventions with clients who have suffered traumatic experiences. One might think at a glance that the painful and disturbing nature of trauma, especially when inflicted in childhood, would be straightforward to tackle in defusion work because it is something that 'happened to the victim from the outside'. In simple terms, clinicians sometimes think this type of experience might be somewhat easier to distance from. However, for us, this view totally misses self as the fundamental basis of fusion and the fact that traumatic experiences typically change the person you see yourself as. Indeed, many victims find it difficult to see themselves as victims, but instead see themselves as weak or even guilty in some way. In this sense, our defusion work with those clients is not about defusing them from what happened to them, but instead defusing them from the painful negative judgments they have about themselves based on what was inflicted upon them. In these cases, it is of paramount importance that the defusion work operates from a safe and stable place where the therapist is almost *inside, rather than outside,* the psychological space of the client. For example, we might say to clients something like this: "I can really understand why you blame yourself for part of this and why other people let you think that way." This safety and validation piece provides an essential foundation for later work on defusion, which simply would not be possible without this because the client would feel misunderstood and unheard. At one level, clients with these experiences must have their perception of their 'guilt' recognized and validated before the internal experiences their trauma generated can be defused.

What we have tried to highlight through the chapter has also been the huge amount of skilled work it takes to separate anyone from their internal experiences, when these experiences hold profound meaning and power over their sense of identity (i.e., when they are fused). For us, defusion means separation, and nothing less than this will qualify as defusion. We would like to put it like this. Weakening the literal meanings of fusion is not defusion. Distinguishing self from one's experience is not defusion. Distancing the self from one's experiences is not defusion. And finally, weakening the behavioral functions of fusion is not defusion. A defused behavioral repertoire will only be achieved when all of these aspects of fusion have been reduced or removed. Defusion can only be said to occur when the self has been freed from the influence of thoughts and feelings and can now be (i.e., respond as) whoever the self wishes to be, irrespective of what they think and feel.

Case analysis Emily: part 2

Recall our client Emily from the beginning of the chapter. After her cancer treatment, she was fused with ongoing health worries and the sense that they made her a burden to her family. As a result, she kept many of her painful internal worries and fears to herself, but then struggled to feel deep connections with the people she loved.

Emily is a good client to use here because after distinguishing her from her internal worries and fears, it might seem that distancing her from these would be a logical next step. However, that would not have worked with this client, nor does it work with other clients with similar experiences. Imagine that you were Emily and had just been through the most frightening experience of your life, where your life actually hung in the balance and you had genuinely faced the real possibility of death. Naturally, you will carry the scar of this in the form of fear and worry for the rest of your life, and partly because death has the potential to become a real possibility sooner than you had anticipated. In this case, it is extremely unlikely that a clinician will be able to establish a workable distance between you and these worries. The reason for this is simple, because they could come true at any time, and you would have to face death. We have been a part of this experience with many clients who have suffered life-threatening illnesses. As a result, we do not engage in any form of distancing with these clients, but that is not to say that we do not do defusion. On the contrary, we try our best to separate these clients from their new identity that is defined by illness and possible death. Hence, similar to the client with chronic pain and the clients with trauma we described above, we work hard to keep these experiences internal and smaller than the person, rather than making them external. And yet, with skill and precision, we can still establish defusion from this place.

Having these recurrent health worries and fears, as well as sharing them, were both highly aversive to Emily. This is understandable. Having worries was frightening because it seemed to bring the pain of death closer to her, and her identity as a living person was thus shattered. Sharing worries with her family filled her with guilt because it made her feel like a bad person because 'she had already caused them enough suffering'. You can now see where the fusion at both levels is in this case. First, worrying about death eroded Emily's identity as alive. Second, being a further burden on her family eroded her identity as a loving family member. While this identification with not being alive and with being a bad relative continue, it is very unlikely that there will be any change in Emily's internal worries or in her sharing of these with her family. This is, therefore, where we targeted our defusion interventions.

Interventions designed to distinguish Emily from her illness and her recurrent worries had worked well. She saw that illness had happened to her unwillingly.

We used the Life as a Journey analogy to emphasize that her illness was a key part of the journey of her life that she had lived thus far. This analogy was central to distinguishing Emily from her worries and fears, because it emphasized that illness was only a part of Emily's identity as a living person, hence reducing the fusion with her identity as a dying person.

Similarly, the analogy allowed us to explore with Emily the whole lifetime of experiences she had shared with her loved ones, again on the great journey of life that she had, including how they had shared her illness with her. As a result, her illness also became part of what the family had experienced together, and thus their shared identity as a family on a journey also contained illness but was not defined by it.

In this way, both aspects of fusion were being reduced.

There was clearly a lot of work to do in reducing the behavioral functions that had become attached to Emily's fusion, especially the hiding of worries and fears from her loved ones. Although the distinction work and the powerful analogy would not have achieved this change in behavior alone, they gave us a good basis for extending this toward behavioral change.

Case analysis Emily: part 3

Using the journey analogy and emphasizing Emily's identity now as a fully living person, we focused on how much she wanted her behavior to be about living (defused identity) versus dying (fused identity).

As a living person, we explored all of the behaviors she could do that were about living, and we questioned together how much she wanted to invest in behaviors that were about dying. Naturally, she wanted to do as much of the former and as little of the latter as possible. Hence, we compiled together a written list of all of her current 'living behaviors' and all of her 'dying behaviors'.

As one might expect, 'buying' into worries about dying and spending time on them was on the list of dying behaviors, as was hiding these worries about death. In contrast, sharing worries and fears was on the living list, as was making plans for holidays, buying a new house, and exploring new ways to be intimate with her husband.

In deactivating the functions of an identity about death and being a bad family member, we were able to weaken fusion at both levels. Furthermore, we activated new functions by attaching them to an identity that was about living, thus ensuring, as much as possible, that fusion would not resurge.

Conclusions

In the final stage of the current chapter, there remains little that we feel we can add to what we have already covered. We hope that we have highlighted that we see defusion as a pivotal piece of psychological wellbeing, and we see defusion interventions as key to achieving this with clients whose identity has been eroded or interrupted by negative experiences, both external and internal. On balance, we wanted to show you how hard fusion is to weaken and the fact that there are places in client's behavioral repertoires where some aspects of defusion interventions cannot weaken fusion. In these cases, you, as an ACT clinician, must make adjustments to your defusion toolkit and find different analogies, metaphors, and exercises to weaken fusion in all of its forms. In this regard, we wish to emphasize again that defusion-based protocols will, in our view, be limited with many clients because they do not allow you to detect fusion correctly and tailor the right aspects of defusion techniques at the right time for your client. On the contrary, working with fusion and defusion creates opportunities for you to be both precise and creative.

References

Espositio, N. J., & Phelton, L. H. (1971). Review of the measurement of semantic satiation. *Psychological Bulletin, 75*, 330–346.

Hayes, S. C. (2005). *Get out of your mind and into your life. The new acceptance and commitment therapy*. Oakland: New Harbinger, pp. 36–37 and 76–77.

Hayes, S. C, Strosahl, K. D., & Wilson, K. (1999). *Acceptance and commitment therapy: An experiential approach to behavior change*. New York: Guilford Press.

Shafran, R., Thordarson, D. S., & Rachman, S. (1996). Thought-action fusion in obsessive compulsive disorder. *Journal of Anxiety Disorders, 10*(5), 379–391.

Titchener, E. B. (1916). *A text-book of psychology*. New York: McMillan, p. 425.

Chapter 4

Creative hopelessness and why it is so central in ACT

Yvonne Barnes-Holmes and Ciara McEnteggart

It makes us very happy to write a chapter on creative hopelessness because we have experienced so many strong emotions and significant positive changes in doing this part of acceptance and commitment therapy (ACT) in our personal lives and with our clients. This chapter will introduce you to creative hopelessness and the very heart of ACT it signifies. We will emphasize throughout how experiencing the intense pain of hopelessness brings us and our clients to the full joy of real and lasting change.

Again, in the interests of clarity and your learning experience, we have divided creative hopelessness interventions into two sections, hopelessness and creativity, which you can follow in your clinical work as a rough sequence. The key components of hopelessness we discuss are: validating change efforts; separating self from change efforts (note the overlap with defusion; see defusion chapter); and undermining change efforts. We will then follow with the critical features of our creativity interventions: accepting responsibility for change; and letting go of the old agenda and beginning anew. But once again, we urge you strenuously not to deliver creative hopelessness in a rigid, stage-like way.

At the beginning and end of the chapter, we again summarize a client, but now we describe someone with whom creative hopelessness interventions were hugely transformative. The chapter contains other real-life client examples and interventions. Again, we have presented personal exercises for you to engage in, in order for you to embrace creative hopelessness with regard to your own efforts to change your internal experiences and the behaviors they drive.

Introduction to creative hopelessness

In terms of the approximate sequence of ACT, creative hopelessness lies between the Contact with Present Moment and Acceptance phases but is essentially nestled within the former. We will argue boldly that creative hopelessness is ACT's centerpiece, around which all other segments must pivot. Indeed, in our view, creative hopelessness is *the* pivotal place within ACT through which all major changes in behavior are facilitated. We have also learned in over 20 years of doing and training

DOI: 10.4324/9781032699691-5

ACT that the ability to fully wrestle with creative hopelessness with oneself and one's clients is the ultimate measure of a good ACT clinician.

It may be obvious to you that creative hopelessness is the combination of the two elements of creativity and hopelessness. Specifically, hopelessness is what we want the client to fully contact about their current efforts to change their internal experiences and especially the behavior driven by them. And creativity is the movement by the client toward a more creative relationship with these experiences that will facilitate new behavior that no longer serves the purpose of changing these experiences (i.e., no longer directed by fusion and avoidance; see defusion chapter). Thus, it goes without saying that a clinician has only established creative hopelessness in a client when *both* of these elements can be experienced. That is, clients must be genuinely hopeless about their current way of living (including changing) and genuinely willing to be creative about finding a new way.

At this early point in the chapter, we feel compelled to acknowledge that the hopelessness you are trying to establish in your clients is extremely painful, disorientating, and at times disheartening for them. Naturally, clients come into therapy with hope for change, but without realizing that change can only come when their verbal system has been largely undermined. Indeed, clients get worse before they get better because the pain they come in with is enhanced by the hopelessness of their current ways of living with this pain and even trying to change it. Delivering this message of hopelessness to clients is *always* agonizing for the ACT clinician too, but we do it because we believe that there is no other way to create lasting change. We will prompt you to recognize and validate this pain, for both clients and yourself as a therapist, throughout the chapter.

We would also like to point out something of a paradox, which you may have already seen above. Although we call this phase of ACT creative hopelessness, the hopeless part actually comes first, followed by the creative part. Again, clients can only get creative about a new way of living after they have contacted genuine hopelessness about their current way. As a result, in the sequencing of the chapter, we cover hopelessness first, followed by creativity. However, in the end, you will see that what has really been established for clients is a type of creative hopelessness.

Case analysis Shaun: part 1

To open the chapter again in a clinically meaningful way, we have summarized below the context of a client with whom our creative hopelessness interventions were pivotal in enabling their problematic behaviors to change in the way they truly wanted. Again, toward the end of the chapter, we revisit this client and summarize the creative hopelessness techniques we used to help them make progress. Shaun was a medical doctor in his 40s. He was socially aloof and quiet, but not cold, in most contexts, including work. The only exception to this was with two close childhood friends, who he believed accepted him entirely for who he was. When he was with either of these individuals, he apparently saw no need to hold back his own views, emotions, or troubles, even if they might seem odd or intense.

In other words, he felt totally at ease around these people, but never with anyone else. At work, he worried constantly about making a mistake, and thus he generally went along with whatever anyone louder than him suggested was "the right way," even if he disagreed with it internally. He then felt frustrated at what he saw as his own "weakness" in this regard.

Shaun had a troubled history with partners. As soon as a woman showed significant affection for him, he started a relationship with her, but none of these lasted more than a few months. Typically, within weeks, he felt a deep, painful longing to be with that partner every minute of the day and was unable to attend to his life fully when the longing was present. Shaun was then needy and intense around his partner, and he became persistently restless about how he might keep her happy.

Shaun had a troubled childhood, which he ironically described as "better than most people's." His mother was an alcoholic who saw him as an inconvenience, while his father worked away a lot. His parents divorced when he was 9 years old, and his mother was awarded full custody. But, whenever his father was nearby, Shaun's mother handed him over as quickly as she could in order to maintain her social life. Similarly, when his father was not working, he found Shaun tiresome to look after and wanted his freedom. Shaun grew up with a sense that his best strategy was to: walk on eggshells around both parents; keep out of their way; cause them no additional trouble; and try to make them love him in any way possible, usually by taking charge of things. Both parents told him regularly that he needed to "man up" and get a grip of his emotions. As a result, Shaun said nothing of his feelings around them and learned to stay distant, calm, and in control of his actions.

Shaun was the couple's second child, they lost a son before he was born. Although this first child died as an infant, his parents were both of the view that he was just the male child they had hoped for. In spite of this professed loss, Shaun saw little evidence of emotional pain or grief by either parent. Because the couple had no further children after Shaun, he lived effectively as their only child.

Shaun had never been to therapy because he believed that it was his responsibility to change his own behavior and get the life he wanted. He desperately wanted: to have more energy; to be able to enjoy life with a wider circle of friends and colleagues; and to express himself better. However, nothing he ever tried seemed to work (e.g., going to the gym, joining social clubs, taking up new hobbies, or embracing new work responsibilities). He fantasized constantly about meeting the "right woman," but felt sure that he would suffocate any relationship with his coldness and a strong need for his own space. Although he referred a lot to his "problematic behavior patterns," he found it difficult to describe them in detail, but reported that he had been trying to "change" them since his early 20s. He also found it extremely difficult to talk about his feelings and simply described everything as "tiredness" and "sadness," both of which he expressed in a rather distant way.

One of his two close friends recently advised Shaun to get therapy because: they saw him less and less; he reported that he no longer loved his job (although this didn't seem true); and he had made no efforts to find a romantic partner in the last

3 years. In Shaun's own words, his "problematic behavior patterns had gotten out of control," and he truly feared more than ever that he would live the rest of his life alone.

You can clearly see that Shaun is very focused on changing himself and how he behaves. Although he truly longs for change, he is unable to articulate what this would look like and why that would matter so much to him. You can also get the impression that Shaun's change agenda may be based on an internal template of how life '*should* be lived' (based on what he learned in his childhood), rather than on what Shaun himself now truly wanted. Shaun's focus on change had clearly allowed him to avoid contacting his own emotions in a deep way. Indeed, one of the changes that he was focusing on was to feel more feelings instead of feeling "nothing." Shaun was clearly in need of creative hopelessness interventions.

Understanding hopelessness

As language-able adults, we have learned what it means to be hopeful about good outcomes and hopeless when these seem impossible to achieve. Creative hopelessness is the same as this but runs deeper. Consider your perspective as an ACT clinician. In the simplest terms, your position toward the client is this – trying to change your internal experiences hasn't and won't work, so it's time to stop. The hopelessness here refers to the high probability that the client's psychological story as it works presently cannot, and will not, allow new behavior to occur. In contrast, it maintains current behavior patterns, even though these are a source of pain and frustration for the client. In short, the functions of behavior (internal experiences and overt action based on them) will not change unless the story itself changes in some way, because it is the story that maintains these functions. As such, *you* can see the trap that clients are in, but they cannot; they are seeking to change internal experiences and behavior inside a system that cannot allow that change.

What hopelessness interventions involve

When beginning to establish hopelessness, you should keep in mind, and emphasize to the client, that you are not challenging the person, but together you are challenging the story and its functions. Once again, establishing hopelessness as a therapeutic aim is far from easy because hope is precisely what clients come to therapy with – hope that you will give them a solution. In the sections below, we will outline the critical features of hopelessness interventions, including: validating change efforts; separating self from change efforts; and undermining change efforts. We will then follow with the critical features of our creativity interventions, including accepting responsibility for change; and letting go of the old agenda and beginning anew.

We do not wish to go any further without explicitly emphasizing a key characteristic that you will need as a clinician when delivering creative hopelessness interventions – *boldness*. We noted above that experiencing hopelessness of all previous change efforts is simply agonizing for you and your clients, and boldness is essential in the face of this acute emotional and professional challenge. You will be tempted to rescue them; let them off the hook by suggesting new behaviors that might work, thus reaching for something akin to behavioral activation. But the true function of this will be to ease your own pain of watching your clients suffer and possible doubts about your professional competence. We totally appreciate your good intentions, but speaking in a strictly functional way, you are throwing a drowning swimmer a stone, whereas if you just hold their hand and stay with them, they will stay afloat and may ultimately be saved.

Validating change efforts

The first and most critical place to start in moving clients toward letting go of hope that surrounds all existing and past efforts to change their internal experiences and the behavior they drive might seem ironic. But it is to validate the very efforts they have made over a long period of time (years or even decades). For example, we have known many clients who have tried different strategies, regimes, and even therapies for 20 or 30 years, and yet their behavior has not changed noticeably. It is particularly important for these clients to validate those enormous, well-intentioned efforts and the inevitability of the position in which they are currently (given their history). But sadly, we have seen so many ACT clinicians who start hopelessness with lists of clients' change efforts that can only make clients feel foolish and stupid. This implicit invalidation runs totally counter to what we want to achieve in hopelessness work, where we aim to validate the person but undermine the story. The box below illustrates how we might offer validation at this first point in hopelessness work, and it is important for you to see just how intense the validation is. For us, validation here works by showing the client that you are on their team *even now*, and that you can understand the rationale and inevitability of their actions without making judgments based on the lack of outcomes. The box below contains an example of the wording we commonly use when making this validation move with clients.

Example of validation of previous change efforts

I have listened carefully and heard all of the things that you've tried to do over a really long period of time, probably even decades. And I have to say that you are a real tryer, and I totally admire you for that.

And I want to be really honest with you and say that if I had been you at any point in that long journey, I would have done exactly the same as you at every turn in that road.

I can see that you put all your efforts into doing what seemed right. You just did what you really had to do, and you did it the best that you could.

And no-one should even try to take that away from you. I certainly would not do that. I really admire you for what you have done, irrespective of where it has led.

One aspect of our hopelessness work, which you may have begun to see already in the validation above, but which will become increasingly visible, is the importance of anchoring *all* of these interventions in the present moment as it exists in the room between the client and you. We cannot emphasize to you enough that clients must begin to get hopeless about their story and its functions *right now*; otherwise, they are still in the story and engaging in the same behavior. If the present moment is not the sole basis for hopelessness, then you cannot guarantee that the old functions attached to the story and its change efforts are being reduced. Even coming into, and being in therapy right now, may be part of those old functions. We will come back to this point again.

Separating self from change efforts

Only after the validation piece above has landed can the client begin to see their change efforts with more distance and less fusion. It is important at this point to explore *all* efforts to change, and to leave no stone unturned in this regard. Before we look at the typical list we formulate with clients, it is important that you understand the rationale for doing this. In technical terms, what we are aiming to do here is to gather all of the clients' change behaviors into a single class of responses that share a single common aim of pushing the client to think, feel, and behave differently. This class of behaviors must become separate from the client without being a source of regret, shame, or judgment, because they are all part of the old story. They just are what that person did, and although they each seemed different at the time, what the client is learning now with you is that they all served the same function. Again, the validation piece here is obvious – the client is not hopeless, but the list is hopeless, although understandable and even admirable.

In the box below, we have provided an example of how we begin to formulate the client's list of change efforts while ensuring that all of the obvious behaviors are included. Specifically, most client lists will include: distraction; positive thinking; avoidance; self-judgment; self-blame; criticism of laziness and lack of motivation; working too hard; working too hard for others; perfectionism; and blaming others. The box below gives examples of each of these types of behavior and it lists for each a common topography that we encounter.

Making the list of change efforts

Now that I can see that you have tried to change for so long and in so many ways, it will really help me to respect those efforts and to fully appreciate what you were trying to do then, if we make a list together. Let's try to include everything that you have done to change the way you think, feel, and act. Let's try to make the list as long as possible and leave nothing out. Everything you tried was worth a shot. So, let's see if we can come up with at least ten things you've done and have a real example of each one.

1. Distraction: I smoke because it calms me down.
2. Positive thinking: I read self-help books and tell myself "it will be okay."
3. Avoidance: I avoid seeing people when I'm feeling down.
4. Self-judgment: I tell myself that "maybe I am not worthy of change."
5. Self-blame: I tell myself "it's all my fault that I got here."
6. Criticism of laziness and lack of motivation: I tell myself "it would be better if I wasn't so lazy and tried harder."
7. Working too hard: I focus on my job because that's what I'm really good at.
8. Working too hard for others: I do my best for my family because they're the best part of my life.
9. Perfectionism: I can't accept any mistakes I make; I have to make things right.
10. Blaming others: I didn't get off to a good start, so I'll never catch up with everyone else.
11. Any other examples...

Once the list is as complete as possible at this point (you may return to it in a later session and can add to the list at any point), we ask the client to reflect now on what it feels like to look at that long list of time, energy, and effort that they invested so heavily in. Typically, at this early point, clients will report a mix of recognition and confusion that they have tried so hard, along with sadness, frustration, and even loss that they invested so much and gained so little. We never try to alter or influence these emotional reactions. Whatever they are, they show that the client is already beginning to see all of their own behaviors on the list as separate from themselves and without self-judgment (remember, judgment would be on the list).

Let's begin to do some personal work in this chapter too. In the box below, we would like you to make your own list of change efforts. As a therapist, you have likely found things that *do* work for you and through which you have genuinely grown as a person, so they can be left out of the list. Thus, your list may well be smaller than a client's at the beginning of therapy. For you, it is crucial that your list contains only the behaviors that you invested in, but which have not resulted in the changes you were hoping for. Please follow the format of our example in the previous box, where you list each type of behavior (e.g., distraction) and then list the topography alongside (e.g., "I smoke because it calms me down").

List of my change efforts exercise

Please write your answers here.

1. Distraction:
2. Positive thinking:
3. Avoidance:
4. Self-judgment:
5. Working too hard:
6. Working too hard for others:
7. Any other examples…

Once you have completed the list, please now write down any emotional reactions that show up *right here and now* as you look at that list. Please ask yourself whether you can be proud of your hard work and effort, even though they have not actually paid off. Remember that at the time you began each effort, you wouldn't have known that it wasn't going to work. You began each new effort in good faith, so it's important to recognize that process while paying less attention to its outcome. As you can see from your own example and that above with clients, the focus here is very much on the genuine intention to change over whether or not this produced the desired outcome. This move might again seem ironic, but it serves to make talking openly about change efforts more appetitive and allows you to orient clients away from things they cannot control and toward things they can (such as their own behavior).

You may have already noticed that we did not build the list of change efforts around experiential avoidance, as many ACT clinicians do. We often hear clinicians present to clients that 'emotional control is the problem'. This appears to assume that emotional avoidance is the dominant, perhaps only, function of a client's change efforts. We think this is a rather simplistic position to adopt because there are multiple functions that any story will acquire, and avoidance is only one of them. The mistake that can easily be made here is two-fold. (1) It suggests that avoidance will reveal itself when the story is challenged, but sadly, we rarely find that things unfold that readily. (2) It implies that behavior will change significantly once avoidance functions are reduced. Again, we often find that this is only part of the solution and far from all of it. In our experience, the concept of "emotional control" doesn't hold much meaning for clients, nor does "avoidance." In order to avoid these mistakes and misunderstandings, we refer to these lists by highlighting the dominant functions they contain, such as "wiping the slate clean," "pretending to be someone else," "taking the pain away," "pretending you're not in pain," and so on. Varying the names we give the list across sessions allows us to share with clients the functions of the behaviors on it.

The example below of one of our clients illustrates how we talk about the list of change efforts. What we want you to appreciate from this client example is the distinction between form and function. All of the "desired" behaviors that the client wanted to engage in were all genuinely good moves for his health and well-being (e.g., eating correctly), and yet he failed to initiate any of these actions for any period of time. Thus, while the topographies of those behaviors were beneficial, the way he was going about starting them had a function that was problematic. For example, he wanted to eat better for some other function than health.

Client example of the impact of making a list of change efforts

A man in his mid-50s with huge professional responsibilities was referred to us for individual therapy. His physical health and well-being had been deteriorating for several years, and he believed that he would soon have a burnout or heart attack. He traveled extensively for work, spending weeks at a time alone in foreign hotels, but reported that he no longer missed his wife or young children. He had a burnout 15 years previously and suggested that 'this might actually be good for him' again, although he believed that the large corporation he managed would punish him for any extended absence. Given his familial responsibilities, he was afraid to take that risk.

He was convinced he could prevent burnout by "getting his act together," which included eating better, exercising more, and meditating more effectively – all (he believed) necessary on a daily basis. He had tried many variations of these desired behaviors, but none lasted more than a day or two. He described himself as lazy and unmotivated for not using his spare time to "look after himself properly," especially given that he was alone so often and had no immediate obstacles to self-care. He had explored every possible avenue of self-improvement he could find, including: diets; exercise regimes; meditation; extended retreats; dozens of self-help books and websites; journaling in many different formats; yoga; pilates; and so on. By the time this client came for help, he was: disgusted by his physical appearance; ashamed about his sensitivity to work stresses; and simply exhausted at his own efforts to change.

This client was hard to validate because he focused much more on outcomes than processes and was blinded by his own sense of failure. The list of his change efforts was obviously focused around physical health and well-being, and he felt strongly that the list be entitled "self-care." However, the moment we named the list self-care, he snorted that this title was further proof of his lack of achievements.

The "self-care" list for this client had 20+ items, each with multiple topographies, and the client spent many days refining it after the session to ensure that "none of his failures went unnoticed." When he returned to session with the newly extended list, he reported that he felt only despair and frustration and that there seemed to be nothing else that he could still try.

Looking at the list was a huge shock for him because it made him feel that only a catastrophic outcome awaited him, like a breakdown or a heart attack. When the therapist asked him to add each of these as "next steps" (the breakdown and the heart attack) to the list, he began to realize that there was something flawed about his strategy, as if these events were clearer evidence that it was too late and that he would have to give up his old ways of trying.

The therapist asked him next if, if he had a breakdown or heart attack, he would surely have more time to eat well and exercise. However, he argued that there would be no point in doing that then because they were part of everything that would have led to those outcomes in the first place. This was a truly creative moment with this client, who then threw the list in the bin and said, "Please let's start again."

At that point, the therapist suggested that the old list be retrieved from the bin and renamed as the "Heart attack list." It was agreed with the client that together they would begin to make a new list (the "Freedom list") across coming sessions. They also agreed to watch out for anything that would match any item on the 'Heart attack list' and ensure that that item had no place on the 'Freedom list'.

Undermining change efforts

It is essential at this point in the hopelessness work to use a number of analogies and metaphors, again to facilitate distance between the client and their own change efforts and to allow them to see them clearly and accurately as separate from themselves (see defusion chapter). Indeed, using analogy and metaphor here also brings something new to the table by gently and metaphorically introducing the idea that none of these efforts have really paid off in the client's life and well-being. This is not a message that could be delivered directly or by instruction because it would simply be too invalidating and would make you aversive as a therapist. You will see the shift here toward a focus on outcomes, where the focus before was more on attempts to change. Again, we want you to recognize that analogy and metaphor used here can begin to undermine the client's former efforts without invalidating them in any way. In the text box below, we have presented what is arguably one of ACT's most well-established metaphors (adapted from Hayes et al., 1999), typically used to begin to undermine a client's previous list of futile efforts to change internal experiences and the behavior attached to them.

The man in the hole metaphor

The situation you are in seems to be a bit like this. Imagine you find yourself in a big field, but you're blindfolded. And all you've been told is that this is how you are supposed to live. But what you don't know and what will make life even harder for you is that the field has some deep, wide holes, and of course, in no time at all, you fall into one. Because you're blindfolded, all you can rely on is feeling around in the darkness with your hands and feet, but still, you can find no escape hatches or gaps that would give you a way out.

Now, when you were first introduced to the field and this way of living, you were given a toolbag, and so you turn now in your desperation to see if there is anything in there that might help you out of this hole. As you feel inside the bag, the only tool your hand recognizes is a small shovel, so you pull that out, with some glimmer of hope that you might be able to do something useful with it. And before long, you find yourself doing the only thing that anyone can do with a shovel, and that's digging. So you dig and you dig and you dig, because at least you're doing something.

But soon you get that sinking feeling that although you're doing your best with what you have, the hole is actually getting deeper; there are still no exits and no gaps. It's soul destroying! All that work and now things are even worse.

So again, you do the only thing you can and you dig and you dig and you dig. Deeper. Faster. With as much effort as you have left. But still, you know that the hole is only getting deeper and deeper.

It's a truly sad situation that you're in here. You're doing everything you can with what you have been given, but life is just getting harder and harder. That's because digging will never get you out of a hole; digging can only make holes bigger. But that's all that anyone can do with a shovel.

We have seen many variations of this amazing metaphor, but sadly, many are too long and too complex. The metaphor's aim here is to gently highlight several features of the client's change efforts to date, and as such, it should not contain or emphasize anything else, lest its key messages be lost. (1) All of the change efforts are similar (all are the same process of digging). (2) The client did everything they could under difficult circumstances (validation of the process). (3) None of these efforts have paid off what the client needed, and in fact, their situation is now worse (outcome). (4) None of these efforts could ever have worked (shovels only make holes bigger, not smaller; hence, that process can never lead to that outcome), but the client couldn't have known that. You can clearly see how the metaphor skillfully, yet gently, emphasizes the futile outcome of everything the client has invested in to change.

What we have also seen ACT clinicians do is to explain the metaphor or very explicitly draw parallels between the client's change efforts and the man in the hole, presumably with the aim of further emphasizing the metaphor's key points. Ironically, however, explanations of analogies and metaphors almost never work, and in fact, these explanations start to feel invalidating, harsh, and even demeaning. As a rule of thumb, if you have to explain a metaphor, it's probably not a good one for that client at that point.

Let's get personal again. In the box below, we would like you to reflect upon your own emotional reactions as you think about your own change efforts as digging. We appreciate that although metaphors make issues feel light and distant, it is still a painful realization that what you have tried in your life so far has not given you the freedom to behave in the way you really want.

Emotional reactions to me as the man in the hole exercise

Please write your answer below

....

....

....

....

Write down any and all of the emotional reactions that show up for you here and now as you think about your own change efforts as digging.

....

....

....

....

....

It's a very sobering place for us as individuals and as therapists to watch our clients make experiential contact in the here and now with the futility of their best efforts. In that sense, all hope for change that way has faded. Notice that we are being very careful with our wording here. We are not saying that all hope is gone (the person is not hopeless); instead, we are saying that all hope of changing through digging is gone. Worse still, we are acknowledging that it was a false hope, because the metaphor illustrates very succinctly that digging to get out of a hole could never have worked.

We are often asked by clinicians how to know when clients are "truly" hopeless. And we typically answer as follows. As a clinician, your job is to begin to separate the client from their futile change efforts and bring them to the realization that none of that behavior will ever produce the outcome they intend for it. That is, hopelessness here doesn't have to be true or complete, as long as it has begun. Clients will still be strongly wedded to or fused with the meaning these change efforts have for them, and that will need more time to loosen. Your job here is just to break the link between efforts to change internal experiences and related behavior (process) and the outcome it promises but can never deliver. In short, no-one can change their internal experiences directly, nor will attempts to do so change any of the behaviors that go with them. Once you begin to break this link, you will already see from a client's face that they are experiencing something challenging, unsettling, and, at times, even profound. If that is the case, you have done good hopelessness work, but you still have more to do in building creativity out of that place.

Once again, it is essential that we put a cautious caveat here. At the beginning of the chapter, we stated that clients get worse before they get better because the pain they come in with is enhanced by the sad realization that their current ways of living and even efforts to change have paid back little. We truly see this with every client with whom our hopelessness work eventually proves to be effective. When hopelessness begins to land, clients can become more anxious, more depressed, more uncertain, more afraid, more needy, and so on. And all of this is understandable and even predictable because perhaps hope in that type of change was the only thing they believed they had left, and now that too is gone. In fact, in clinical terms, it is worth seeing these downturns in mood and behavior as something like an extinction burst. Ironically, they may be evidence that you have actually challenged the old agenda. So, while we recognize that this will feel like a very scary and uncertain place for you to be as a therapist (when the client seems to be getting worse), we would simply say: be bold; hang tight; and stay in the room with yourself and your client. The next step, beyond hopelessness, is creativity.

Understanding creativity after hopelessness

Creativity here is the movement by the client toward a more creative relationship with their internal experiences and the behavior they drive, including all of the behaviors of trying to change these experiences. In this section, you will see that what we are referring to is not creativity in the generic sense, but more a space that opens up once the hopelessness of old change efforts has been fully experienced. That is, where hopelessness opens up space and the possibility for genuine change, the next creative piece shows how that space can be filled and how new behavior can thrive.

What creative hopelessness interventions involve

Creative hopelessness interventions should never be forced or driven by the therapist; they should not look like behavioral activation. This part of the work needs time for old functions to weaken and for genuinely new functions to begin to be established. In the sections below, we will outline the critical features of creative hopelessness interventions, including: accepting responsibility for change; and letting go of the old agenda and beginning anew.

Accepting responsibility for change

An important distinction that we often make with clients when doing creative hopelessness work is between blame and responsibility, particularly with regard to how they ended up where they did (failed outcomes). A little verbal trick that ACT clinicians use frequently is to alter the word "responsibility" to "response-ability" (i.e., the ability to respond). This small technique is useful here because in a gentle validating way, it allows the client to own the outcomes of their digging. That is, they were able to respond, and they did so by digging. You can see that this has a neutrality to it that blame does not, because blame is more negative and outcome-focused. If we take this one step further and add that clients were able to respond before and did so by digging, then clients are now able to respond again but no longer want to do so by digging. You can easily see the self-empowerment that begins to emerge and how this seems genuinely creative. The simple distinction you are making is this. *Then*, you were able to respond before, and you dug, and that produced this terrible outcome. *Now*, you are able to respond again, and if you don't dig, you can produce a very different outcome. It will be clear to you that this distinction is empowering but not directive or instructive.

With clients who are particularly prone to self-judgment, we further unpack the disadvantages and harshness of blame versus response-ability. ACT clinicians have long used the addition in the text box below to give clients distance on their own, often automatic self-judgments. You will see that it is merely a brief extension of the Man in the hole metaphor.

The what blame looks like metaphor

Let's just take an honest look here and now at how you have blamed yourself since you came through my door today and how it looks to me. I just sit here and watch you stand at the edge of the deep hole in that field that you fell into. And you look down at yourself, wet, tired, and desperate, at the bottom of that hole. And then, in an instant, I see you throwing dirt on top of your own body and shouting abusively, "How did you get in here you idiot?" And of course, I can see from here how that is working, and as I look down at you in that hole, I know that that's really the last thing that will help you in there. I can see immediately that the person in the hole just got weaker, more frightened, and more alone. So, if this is really about helping you to get yourself out of that hole, even though you did dig yourself into part of it, I simply ask you, will that really help?

And, let me also ask you this rather intrusive and perhaps painful question. If that was your son or your daughter or your partner, is that what you would really do, if you found them lying in a hole, even if they had dug themselves into it. No, I suspect not. It seems as if that level of judgment and cruelty is only reserved for you.

This brief extension of the Man in the hole metaphor that unpacks blame, especially self-blame with regard to the poor outcomes of previous change efforts, is very powerful and often emotional. This emotional aspect of it allows clients to see that blame often feels as if it will facilitate behavior change, but because it drains energy and power and is largely demoralizing, it actually has the opposite effect. The short shift in perspective-taking at the end also serves to highlight the cruelty of self-blame and how that too is unlikely to support change.

Let's get personal again. In the box below, we would like you to reflect upon your own change efforts and whether you are able to accept response-ability for changing each item on your list.

Response-ability for change exercise

Please write your answer below.

....

....

....

....

....

....

Take a look at your list of change efforts. For each item, we would ask you to do two things.

1. Notice that this was what you did before.
2. Now, ask yourself would you do it again.

....

....

....

....

....

....

....

....

Letting go of the old agenda and beginning anew

In order to fully experience hopelessness, clients can do one of two things. They can accept response-ability for every time they pick up the shovel; contact the cost of each and every one of these times; and commit to not doing this again. Or, they can keep convincing themselves that it might eventually work and keep digging. At least now they have a choice, which they didn't have before when they were just being blindly led by their story (this is the creative part). Getting to a place where the client can clearly see the choice between these two options and where they can fully feel the weight of the damage of digging as one of these options is a critical aim of our hopelessness work. We often present the following adaptation of the Chinese handcuffs metaphor (the original metaphor is from Eifert & Forsyth, 2005) as a way of highlighting the response-ability and cost pieces to clients. Notice carefully how the end of the metaphor offers a clear choice of behaving in a new (creative) way that is different from the old agenda.

The Chinese handcuffs metaphor

(The finger traps are physically present)

Take a look at these little Chinese handcuffs, I show them to lots of clients. Because I see so many situations that are just like this.

So, how they work is that you insert each index finger into each end of the straw and push in as far as you can. [Client pushes in]

And when you get really far in, now try to pull each finger back out. [Client tries to pull out]

Can you feel how tight the straw is now around each finger? And when you feel that tightness, what's the first thing you'd like to do? [Client usually says 'pull out harder']

Exactly. The more trapped we feel, the harder we want to get out of that trap. It's like an instinct to get out. So, why not just try to do that, really try actively this time. [Client tries to pull out]

So, where has that gotten you now? [Client usually says 'more stuck']

Exactly. And it's a little scary, isn't it?

So, now you're really stuck, and just like being the man in the hole with the shovel, you have done some of this to yourself and you can honestly take response-ability for that.

But, now let's see if we can go somewhere else with this painful trap you have found yourself in. What if instead of doing the obvious instinctive thing and trying to pull your fingers back out, you did the very opposite thing and pushed into your fear, instead of pulling away from it?

What do you think would happen? Try it and see. [Client pushes fingers in and straw loosens]

Isn't that surprising? Of course, you have been doing what everyone would do and running for the hills when you feel trapped and the fear shows up. But if you don't let fear move your fingers for you, and you actually choose to move them for yourself, then what happens is that you actually get what you want, as much as that's available. Maybe you won't get completely out of there, but any freedom is better than none.

What if we say your life now at this age is like you having been in handcuffs for years and years, and the reality is that 100% freedom is no longer an option for you, even if you pushed in all the time? Let's think about that now. If you're 45 years old, married with children, and have a demanding job, it's probably true that you have about 40% of freedom still available to you. So, some freedom is gone, some by accident, and some by choice. Either way, it's gone forever. So, your fingers are in a tighter place than a few years ago, and no matter how hard you pull, you will never again be totally, 100% free. So your fingers have lost 60% freedom; they'll never be out of the trap, but things could be a lot worse. They could be much tighter. They still have 40% of the total freedom they once had.

So, now what will you do as you live your life with that 40%?

Will you pull hard against it, convincing yourself you'll get 100% back?

Or will you push right into that 40% knowing that it's your best bet, and trying your hardest every day to get 100% of 40%, rather than pulling back and only getting 50% of 40%?

That's your choice now.

Although the metaphor above is long, it is carefully sequenced, with each part having its own clear message. (1) All of the client's change efforts are costly (this undermines the old agenda). (2) Leaning into pain seems counterintuitive but can give space (this adds a new function of leaning in). (3) The client contacts the reality of their losses (adding strength to the new function of leaning in). (4) The client is asked to be willing to lean into the place they are now in their lives in order to avoid further loss (separates old functions from new function of leaning in). You can clearly see how the metaphor skillfully and gently emphasizes the difference between the old change agenda and a new (creative) one.

Let's get personal again. In the box below, we would like you to reflect upon your own losses and how much freedom you are left with in your life as a whole.

The 'How much freedom do you have left to play with?' exercise

Please write your answer below.
Reflect on all of the losses that accrued from your change efforts and ask yourself the following:

1. What % of my life did this cost me?
2. What % of my freedom do I have left?
3. What do I want to do with the % I have left?

....

....

....

....

....

....

What you want clients to really face at this point in creative hopelessness is the fact that they have a simple choice: the old way or the new way. It's not so much about what the new way will look like, but more about *completely* undermining the old way. If you do that, the new way, in whatever topography it comes, will be naturally appetitive. Indeed, at this point, we would caution you strongly not to push or bombard clients with new ways. Instead, keep things simple here, so that they don't get confused or overwhelmed and thus get pulled back into the old change agenda. This simplicity is perfectly illustrated by the old ACT metaphor called the tug-of-war with the monster (found in Hayes et al. (1999)).

The tug-of-war with the monster metaphor

Your situation here reminds me of being in a tug-of-war with a monster. A big, ugly, strong monster. In between you and the monster is a pit, and as far as you can tell, it is bottomless. If you lose this tug-of-war, you will fall into this pit, and your life will be over. So you pull and pull, but the harder you pull, it seems, the harder the monster pulls. And, it appears that you are edging closer and closer to the pit.

The hardest thing to see is that your job here is not to win the tug-of-war. Your job is to drop the rope.

This metaphor is one of ACT's simplest. But, when delivered as a physical metaphor, it is hugely powerful and transformative. The rope represents all previous change efforts, and the physical act of loosening that imaginary rope from a client's hand feels like a real act of closure. The metaphor points clearly to this as the only way forward in the context of an unwinable war with a monster and a bottomless pit.

Case analysis Shaun: part 2

Recall our client Shaun from the beginning of the chapter, who despised himself for what he saw as a pathetic inability to stand up for himself and be his own man. Notice the overlap between this ongoing harsh self-judgment and the echoes of Shaun's parents demanding that he "man up." Notice also that the harder he tried to man up, the weaker and more needy he seemed to become around others, especially intimate partners. Shaun's way of managing this dilemma was to be quiet and aloof or intense and needy, both of which were behavioral patterns he was drawn toward, ashamed of, and unable to break. Although clearly hopeless and exhausted by these relentless efforts, Shaun was unable to describe any of his feelings in detail, another "deficit," of which he had shame and hopelessness.

It took almost ten sessions for the female therapist to really get to know Shaun. During this time, there were few emotional conversations, and he stared quietly into space much of the time, nodding his head at what the therapist suggested. When she got close to any sore topics, such as his childhood or intimate relationships, it felt as if Shaun left the room emotionally. He then criticized himself for "being avoidant." When he eventually appeared safe and comfortable in the therapeutic relationship, the therapist began to address this 'switching off'.

Shaun began these conversations with strong judgments that 'switching off is weak'. He was heavily fused with this as his failing and responsibility and did not easily see it as historical inheritance linked to coping with harsh parents. Neither did he see the judgment of weakness as identical to what his parents said repeatedly. Contrary to those judgments, the therapist portrayed switching off as 'strong, calm, collected and reflective of a smart child'. This was not delivered or presented explicitly as a type of cognitive disputation; it was gently designed to make talking about switching off more appetitive and to loosen the negative judgments around it (defusion). This was combined with discussions about how it was natural that Shaun's parents saw this behavior as weak, yet it could also be viewed as a strong survival strategy. A key rationale of these sessions was to open up the dialogue to include Shaun's fusion with the story "I am a weak man" and the relentless self-change efforts that were functions of that story. The therapist also compassionately emphasized how existing behaviors (e.g., over-eating and being needy with partners) are inevitable collateral that come with struggling with a harsh, painful, fused story about being weak.

You can see how this defusion work was essential to help the therapist get inside the story about being weak, where the functions that Shaun was trying to tackle directly but unsuccessfully were located. Note that this was precisely where hopelessness was targeted, rather than targeting hopelessness directly at the 'failed' behaviors themselves, because Shaun's hopelessness and frustration there were actually part of the problem and not part of the solution.

The therapist openly presented the "I am weak" story as hopeless because if Shaun's parents and Shaun have already deemed him weak in many aspects of his life so far, then "perhaps you are weak, so why fight it, surely fighting it only seems to make you weaker and weaker." This is a delicate and painful track to take and may seem counterintuitive, but this is the exact place where Shaun was stuck and alone. It was a place he hid desperately from others, and thus it was essential that the therapist sit inside that hopeless place with Shaun. Shaun became deeply emotional at the finality of these discussions and the deep sense that 'his weakness had already been decided upon by his parents and by himself'. This was the first time Shaun was truly emotional. He described his main emotions as sadness that this was really true and fear that he would never be able to change it. The hopelessness of the weakness story was very obvious at this point, and the validation move by the therapist had worked well. Shaun reported that he felt close to the therapist but not needy, and that he was proud of the emotions he felt and his courage in sharing them with a woman.

In the description of the dialogue and interventions above, you can see the various pieces of the hopelessness work in terms of validating change efforts, separating self from change efforts, and indirectly undermining change efforts.

Shaun was then presented with a choice – playing the past-tense parental game where his weakness has already been decided upon and which was not winnable, or trying to achieve what he really wanted for himself. The latter was positioned as a 'strong move, no matter what the outcome'. Shaun felt a deep sense of response-ability and ownership over the choice and quickly felt free and empowered to act in new ways. This was a truly creative space in which he could accept his past and yet create a "new and different" future. Shaun loved the idea of choosing, but also saw that there was no longer a need to rush or achieve any of this quickly. He embraced the idea that his life was a journey dominated thus far by his parents' story about him being weak, but the next steps of his journey would be his own, and thus, by definition, they would be strong. This was clear evidence that Shaun accepted responsibility for change, but without pressure, and had let go of the old agenda.

Conclusions

Creative hopelessness is the central ingredient of ACT, around which all other components revolve. Willingness and ability to tolerate the struggle inherent to creative hopelessness, both in yourself and in your clients, are necessary for good practice in ACT.

This component of ACT is the combination of the two elements: creativity and hopelessness. Clients need to be fully in touch with the unworkability of their behavior and the hopelessness of continuing to invest in the same strategy before they can move to creativity. The movement toward a more creative relationship with painful experiences requires that behavior is no longer driven by fusion and avoidance. Creative hopelessness is achieved only when clients can be genuinely hopeless about their current way of life *and* must be genuinely willing to find a new creative way.

Inducing hopelessness in your clients is often very painful for therapists because they are eager to help and do not want to cause them additional pain. However, it has been our experience that there is no other way to create lasting change.

In over 20 years of doing and training ACT, we have witnessed many changes in the world of ACT. One change has particularly affected and saddened us: the diminishing importance of creative hopelessness. We increasingly see new ACT clinicians gloss over or even totally ignore this fundamental element of the work. In clinical, experiential, and functional terms, we find it beyond baffling how this situation could have emerged and how anyone can believe that they are truly doing ACT without creative hopelessness being at the center of their clinical rationale and interventions. ACT without creative hopelessness is like smiling without a sense of joy or eating without a sense of taste. As a clinician, if you are not using creative hopelessness as the main axis and pivot of your work, you are, in our opinion, not doing ACT, and your client's need and desire for real change have much less hope of ever coming true.

References

Eifert, G. H., & Forsyth, J. P. (2005). *Acceptance and commitment therapy for anxiety disorders: A practitioner's treatment guide to using mindfulness, acceptance, and values-based behavior change strategies*. Oakland, CA: New Harbinger, pp. 146–149.

Hayes, S. C., Strosahl, K., & Wilson, K. G. (1999). *Acceptance and commitment therapy: An experiential approach to behavior change*. New York: Guilford Press.

Chapter 5

Learning to stay
in the here-and-now

Marjolein Vleugel

In this chapter, I will discuss working in the present moment, also known as working in the here-and-now. Therapists are trained to listen and respond to our clients' stories. By definition, these stories are not anchored in the present moment. They usually refer to the client's past or future. This focus on the past and/or future makes these stories challenging to influence, as behavior can only be changed in the here-and-now.

I will first delve into what I mean by the here-and-now in process-based acceptance and commitment therapy (ACT) and how it encompasses more than just practicing mindfulness. You will learn why we are easily pulled away from the here-and-now and why it is difficult to remain in the present moment. This challenge applies not only to the client but also to you as the therapist. I will teach you how to cultivate the ability to "be in the here-and-now" because it is a skill that can be learned and familiarized with, enabling you to apply it in your work with clients. Being in the here-and-now is a skill that can become a fundamental attitude applicable in every interaction. Additionally, you will learn when *not* to work in the here-and-now. Overall, the here-and-now helps you to move not just from your head but also from your experience (your heart) and your feet. After reading this chapter, you will understand that working in the here-and-now is an essential skill in your clinical practice because it is from this point that we can truly make progress.

Throughout this chapter, I will provide case examples and exercises to give you a clear understanding of this challenging work. Although various components of ACT may overlap in a therapy session, I will separate them as much as possible for the purpose of this chapter.

Case Margaret: part 1

Margaret has come into therapy and seeks help for symptoms such as flashbacks, hyper-vigilance, difficulty concentrating, muscle pain, trembling, and feeling overheated. These symptoms are so severe that whenever they occur, she does nothing but lie in bed. Margaret wants to get rid of her symptoms, or as she puts it: "I want my life back, I want to be the way I used to be and do what I always did."

DOI: 10.4324/9781032699691-6

She spends her days at home and hardly engages in any enjoyable activities like walking or going out to eat because she's afraid her symptoms will flare up. Every time I try to address Margaret's symptoms, she starts talking about how she wants to function as she used to. She goes into detail about all the things she can no longer do due to her symptoms, saying things like: "When the pain in my muscles decreases, I can start walking again" or "When I no longer experience flashbacks, I can go out to eat with my family," and "If only I hadn't chosen this line of work, I wouldn't have these symptoms." These are signals that Margaret struggles to stay in the here-and-now.

What do we mean by the here-and-now?

Mindfulness is not the same as here-and-now work

When I first learned about ACT, I was taught that the here-and-now was the same as mindfulness. I learned various mindfulness exercises such as "The Breathing Space," "Leaves on a Stream," and "The Body Scan." I practiced them for myself, then did these exercises with my clients and assigned them as homework. Clients often found doing these exercises in a session enjoyable. They reported feeling calmer, having fewer thoughts, and feeling better overall. Many clients quickly concluded that practicing mindfulness exercises helps you feel better.

However, I also noticed that some clients had fewer positive experiences. Some shared that they had tried mindfulness before and that it wasn't for them; they felt too restless or believed they could never succeed at it. It's not uncommon to have both positive and negative experiences with mindfulness. When you read information about mindfulness on the internet or in magazines, it often gives the impression that practicing mindfulness leads to positive outcomes, such as:

- Being free from thoughts
- Feeling good
- Not being bothered by unpleasant emotions
- Knowing exactly what you want.

It would be wonderful if all of that were true and if every mindfulness exercise resulted in such positive experiences. If these benefits were a consequence for everyone, everyone would be practicing mindfulness. Unfortunately, the reality is different. Looking at my own experience, I know that doing mindfulness exercises is not always pleasant and enjoyable. I rarely have moments without any thoughts, and there have been plenty of times when it made me feel more restless and impatient.

We often jump to the conclusion that doing mindfulness exercises will make our problems disappear. While that can indeed be a result, it is certainly not always the case. When we literally pause, as in a mindfulness exercise, the experience may be that our minds are filled with thoughts, or we encounter restlessness and unpleasant emotions, which may even intensify. Sometimes, we may become more confused instead of having a clear sense of what we want to do. If you expect your experience to be positive and it is not, you might quickly assume that you are doing something wrong or that there's something wrong with *you*.

So, are mindfulness exercises (or so-called attention exercises) bad to use? Not at all. These exercises were helpful for me personally and as a therapist, and they still are. It is essential, however, to understand the purpose for which we use mindfulness. Mindfulness serves a very different purpose than striving for peace in your mind and in your life. These exercises are highly effective for training your attention to be in the here-and-now as a continuous process. It's about noticing where your attention is right now, in this moment. Recognizing where you are, in the here-and-now, which might even be an unpleasant place. It involves feeling what you feel in and on your body, experiencing your emotions and thoughts, whether positive or negative. Hearing the sounds, smelling the scents, sensing the temperature – in short, experiencing what is present now, regardless of whether the experience is positive or negative. This is a fundamental difference from the notion that mindfulness is about striving for something positive or achieving a positive state as the end result. Being in the here-and-now is about observing and following the process rather than aiming for a specific (positive) outcome.

Being present with what is happening

Being present and being in the here-and-now in a session with your client means noticing. Moment to moment, you observe what is happening within yourself, with the client, and between both of you. When you are in conversation with a client, the client responds to what you say or do. As a result of your behavior, something happens with the client. It triggers a reaction, a thought, or a feeling. The client responds with their body, saying something, or remaining silent. This behavior, in turn, triggers something in you. And this cycle continues, creating an interaction between you, which is also referred to as the therapeutic relationship.

You can liken this process to a dancing couple. Together with your client, you are dancing. When you take a step, it prompts the client to move as well. This behavior from the client then sets something in motion within you, leading to your next movement, and the cycle continues, back and forth. And thus, a shared dance emerges.

In this interaction with your client, not only does the client respond to your behavior, but you also respond to your behavior. For example, what you say to your client might evoke thoughts in your mind like, 'Oh, why did I say something so silly?' or 'That was a good question from me.' The client experiences similar inner reactions. Everything they do also triggers something within them. In essence, the step you take in your dance not only influences the client but also shapes your subsequent steps. It's the same for the client – their steps influence their next moves. In reality, there are three dances occurring: one within you, one within the client, and one between both of you.

This presence, this complete connection with yourself, your client, and what unfolds between you, is always present. Sometimes it's more prominent and explicit, while other times, it might be less obvious and in the background. However, it is always there. We don't see working in the here-and-now as an activity to be done and then completed, like a mindfulness exercise with a clear beginning and end. In our work, here-and-now work is ongoing. It is a fundamental attitude of the therapist and the foundation of how we work. Whether you are working with self-as-content, defusion when someone becomes fused with their thoughts, or doing values work, the here-and-now component is continuous throughout. It is embedded in the therapist's attitude and interventions.

As a therapist, observing and following behavior happens in a moment-by-moment manner, allowing us to see how the client dances with you. We are continuously dancing, with each topic, in every session, from the beginning to the end of therapy. Consequently, we are constantly aware of what is happening with ourselves, what is happening with the client, and what is happening between us. I can understand if you are thinking, "Wow, that's a lot to observe." I can't deny that I feel the same way. Engaging in conversations in this manner, where you are in the here-and-now, can be intense, but it has helped me to get to know my own dance better. I now have a better understanding of which steps I take when, which allows me more space to see the client's behavior and what unfolds between us. This is why we cannot emphasize enough the importance of undergoing personal therapy or experiential work where you can get to know your own dance well in order to perform this process-based work effectively.

Why is it challenging for both the client and the therapist to stay in the here-and-now?

Now that you know what the here-and-now means, it does not necessarily mean it is easy to achieve. As humans, we are constantly preoccupied with the future. We think about what we want to do tonight or this weekend, what we need to do to get fit or lose weight. We constantly set goals, both in our personal lives and in our work. Think about all the bucket-list books that are circulating, where we can freely fantasize about what we still want to achieve and where we want our lives to go. Or consider the reason why you are reading this book – perhaps because you want to learn more about process-based ACT or become a better therapist.

This tendency is entirely normal and happens continuously. Even as I write this, my thoughts wander to the future – what we will have for dinner tonight, whether I need to buy groceries for it, when I will do that, and so on. When I have these thoughts, I cannot write. They pull me away from the writing process, from the here-and-now. To be able to write, I need to direct my attention to the here-and-now. In the following paragraphs, I will show you that many factors influence the tendency to be pulled away from the here-and-now.

'Living there-and-then' keeps us away from the here-and-now

From a very young age, it is ingrained in us that it is essential to focus on the future, on 'there-and-then.' My parents used to tell me when I was young that I should finish my plate because it would make me big and strong in the future. They encouraged me to do well in school because that would lead to high grades and a bright future. They also promised me a cookie if I got dressed quickly and said we would go playing on the swing later that afternoon if I sat still now. Notice how often we use 'if … then' constructions in our language and how often we are preoccupied with the future.

Being concerned with there-and-then has its advantages. The nice thing about 'there-and-then thinking' is that it provides a sense of predictability and, consequently, a kind of certainty. This feeling arises when the predictions made for the future come true. When we receive that promised cookie after getting dressed or go playing on the swing after sitting still, as planned. Being focused on the future, on there-and-then, helps make the world seem more manageable and controllable.

From a young age, we learn that there's a there-and-then, and that it's important to be concerned with it because there-and-then appears more organized, predictable, and better. After all, there-and-then thinking suggests that in the future you will be big and strong, get good grades, life will be good, you will get treats, do enjoyable things, and you know what you need to do to get there. The problem is that when we learn that there-and-then is better, we indirectly conclude that being in the here-and-now is apparently not as good.

When this continuous relationship between prediction and outcome is repeatedly emphasized and confirmed, we stop recognizing it as a prediction. We forget that predictions might have different outcomes. There-and-then thinking creates the illusion of knowing what will happen and, from there, the idea that you know what you should do now to achieve that outcome. We do this so often because it gives us confidence, security, and a feeling of control, to the extent that we no longer realize we are doing it. Because we are unaware of this 'there-and-then thinking,' it becomes challenging to do something different, such as being in the here-and-now and seeing it for what it is – an idea of how the future might be, rather than an accurate prediction of reality.

So far, we have only given examples related to the future. However, we also indulge in 'there-and-then thinking' about the past. How often do we say things like: "If only I had tried harder back then, things would have turned out better for me," or "If that person hadn't done that to me, I wouldn't have these problems now." Perhaps these statements are true to some extent – you could have done better, or someone did something to you – but we will never know if things would have been better for you or if you wouldn't have had any problems now. These predictions or expectations of the future might also come true. However, this is not about whether something is true or not.

The crucial aspect is that we anchor and fixate our 'self' in there-and-then. We view ourselves from the perspective of there-and-then, as if we were already there and not in the here-and-now. Consequently, we act more on an image of ourselves from the perspective of there-and-then than from our actual selves here-and-now.

Regularly pausing to consider the questions in the following short exercise can help you notice how often you are living in there-and-then.

> **Take a moment to notice exercise**
>
> Take a moment now to notice where you are. Are you in the here-and-now? Or are your thoughts already wandering to there-and-then? Take a few minutes to observe what's happening, where your attention is.

Maybe you noticed that you were already thinking about how this information could help you as a therapist. Or perhaps you managed to keep your attention on your experiences in the here-and-now until it was drawn away again to something from the past or the future. We all easily get pulled away from the here-and-now. Again, that's not a problem; it's simply what happens. It's nice and helpful to be able to think about how we want to approach situations in the future, and it's also nice and helpful to be present in the here-and-now.

We are very well trained in being preoccupied with there-and-then and significantly less skilled at being present in the here-and-now. This makes it more challenging to switch positions: from there-and-then to here-and-now. This pattern is not only prevalent in our daily lives as human beings but also, particularly, as therapists.

The influence of training

During my basic training as a psychologist in the 1990s and later during my training as a healthcare psychologist, I learned to listen to the client's complaints and talk with the client about these issues. The client presented their complaints, and I had to determine which classification these complaints fit into, how they originated, and then tell the client (often based on a protocol) what they could do to make the complaints disappear. Only if this were successful, I thought, would I be a good therapist.

I worked this way for a long time. You could say that I learned to look at what kind of dance the client was performing, how they could learn to dance better, or make fewer missteps to win more beautiful prizes (i.e., feel better). In other words, therapy focused on the client's complaints and was primarily aimed at achieving a better outcome, a more beautiful prize. It sounds logical, and many of you likely practice therapy this way. It is how we've been taught to act. We are focused on achieving a better outcome (there-and-then). This expectation is also present among clients, employers, health insurers, etc. Our eyes are fixed on the idea that it will be better there-and-then, and we have now learned that when we focus on there-and-then, we are not present in the here-and-now.

However, to achieve a different outcome there-and-then, we need to know what we are doing here-and-now – that is, "what steps are we actually taking?" When we only look at there-and-then, we do not get a comprehensive view of the whole story as discussed in Chapter 2. But that is easier said than done because we are all trained to look specifically at there-and-then.

The influence of language

In addition to our training, the use of language and our familiarity with it is also a factor that takes us out of the here-and-now. How we deal with language is like a fish swimming in water. The fish hardly notices that it is in water; it just swims. Likewise, we are so accustomed to using language that we do not even realize that language is something we do. We barely notice how much influence language has on us; we simply use it. While it is great that we have language at our disposal, it also allows us to move away from the here-and-now.

The following example, which I share with participants in almost every ACT training, is about our dog, Pebbles. The first time I heard a version of this metaphor was in a workshop with Dermot Barnes-Holmes.

Pebbles metaphor

We have a dog, and her name is Pebbles. Pebbles sleeps a lot but also enjoys roaming around our garden. Sometimes, we forget that she's outside, even when it's raining. Although our dog loves swimming, she doesn't like being outside in the rain. How do you think Pebbles reacts when we let her inside? Exactly, the poor thing wags her tail, settles into her bed, and starts licking herself dry. … Now, imagine the same thing happening to my husband, where he stands outside a closed door in the rain. How do you think he will react when he is let in?

People are often caught up in their thoughts through language, which takes them away from direct experience. They no longer notice the changes in their immediate experience. Consequently, they also do not act based on that experience but rather on the story in their minds. Dogs are much more (probably always) in the here-and-now than us humans. The dog is "happy" and "content" because it is now in a situation, indoors and dry, where it feels comfortable. When this situation changes from outside to inside, she's content. On the other hand, my husband will undoubtedly have various thoughts about the situation. Thoughts like "Why won't they let me in?" or "Why don't they see me?" or "I'm always being excluded." You can imagine that these thoughts evoke a negative or even angry feeling. These thoughts and feelings are also present here-and-now within my husband. However, when he enters inside, he will most likely act based on those thoughts and not on his experience of entering a warm, dry space. By not noticing this latter experience and not directing his attention to it, it does not play a role in his behavior. If it did, he would undoubtedly be grateful to us for letting him in.

Being in the here-and-now is about seeing what is happening, being present with everything that is. Noticing that we have these thoughts and the accompanying feelings. Observing the situation, that you are outside in the rain. Realizing that you would like to be inside. Experiencing the angry or negative thoughts that arise. And noticing that people are letting you in, where it is warm and dry.

When we get carried away with stories like "Why won't they let me in? Why don't they see me? I'm always being excluded," we drift away from other experiences that are also present at that moment, and we may miss important information. For example, the pleasant experience of being let inside. Language easily takes us away from the here-and-now, causing us to think about the dance we want, instead of experiencing the steps we are taking at that moment. As a result, our thinking mostly guides our behavior, and we hardly allow our direct experience to play any role.

It's difficult to stay with pain

Apart from the fact that we rarely learn to look at the individual steps of the dance, these steps can also be very painful and confronting. It can feel more pleasant to quickly move on with the dance, rather than looking at, staying with, and experiencing the impact of each individual step. Most people do not like being close to pain and discomfort. We all have a natural tendency to move away from discomfort and pain. It simply feels more attractive to move away from it, to be in the realm of there-and-then.

This applies not only to clients but also to us as therapists. This is why we often say, "Everything will be okay," without even knowing whether something will or will not turn out well. We shift our focus to the future instead of staying with the pain. Staying with it, so that we can experience and explore it. Some clients come to therapy with the request to get rid of what they consider to be bad or undesirable behavior. Other clients experience their current behavior as unpleasant and fear it may become even worse in the future. As humans, we tend to focus on how things can be better and different, and we prefer not to dwell on what we are currently doing and the reasons behind it because that can be too painful to look at.

I expect you can recognize this in yourself. For instance, when we discover something about ourselves that we do not like, we tell ourselves that we must try a little harder to be the exact opposite. When I tell myself that I am not good enough, it immediately leads to the thought that I must do all sorts of things to become good enough. The story of "not being good enough" prompts me to take steps toward working hard, doing a lot, and taking action. When I take those steps (working hard, doing a lot), my attention is focused on wanting to be a better version of myself, a version that is good enough in the future. I move away from the here-and-now, from the version that is not good enough. Although working hard and doing a lot may give me a good feeling in the short term, they do not make the thoughts of not being good enough disappear from my life. Every time these thoughts arise in me, I engage in the same kind of dance. The frustrating part is that these thoughts do not disappear from my life because of this dance.

Working in the here-and-now has helped me look at the steps I am making in the dance. I tell myself that I am not good enough. It is painful to see that. Painful to experience that it is me, who says this to myself and no one else. By learning to look at this painful step, daring to look at it, I have learned to see what my next step often becomes. This, too, is painful and confronting. The realization that I am the one taking these steps. That I am the one doing this. That I am the one moving in a direction where I don't actually want to go. And yet, I do it.

Changing the perspective from there-and-then (quickly dancing through) to here-and-now (pausing to examine each step) allows us to see what is truly happening in this moment. Being in the here-and-now is not necessarily a better position; it is just a perspective, similar to there-and-then. It is a perspective from which we are not accustomed to acting. For many of us, it is a relatively new behavior.

Working in the here-and-now, how do you do it?

In process-based ACT, we focus on the steps the dance takes. The prize to be won is that you can move in a direction where you truly want to go. While keeping that prize in mind, the focus is on the dance itself. What steps are you taking now? What causes you to stumble? If you stumble, what do you experience? What step do you take then?

Not being in the here-and-now is a bit like living in the hustle and bustle of daily life. You wake up, go to work, walk the dog, cook, clean, exercise, raise the children, and before you know it, one day you wake up, you are 75 years old, and you realize that your life has passed you by without you even noticing. You wonder, "How did I end up here?" It's like riding a rollercoaster with your eyes closed. We miss parts of our experiences when we do not learn to be present in the here-and-now. There are several different ways to learn to open our eyes, such as slowing down, allowing active silences, and changing our posture.

Slowing down is crucial

To see and experience what is happening in the here-and-now, it is important to learn to slow down. Compare it to different ways of reaching a destination. For example, you can take the car or walk. Taking the car will probably get you to your destination faster. But if you walk, it will take more time, and you can see more along the way. While walking, you can notice how the surroundings affect you, and you can notice what you need at that moment and act accordingly.

In process-based ACT, we focus on looking at and exploring the journey, rather than trying to reach the destination as quickly as possible. Speed often comes at the expense of realizing how we arrived at our destination. Learning to look at the journey makes us more aware of which turns we can and want to take, when we can keep going, when we need to rest, whether we are still on the right track, or if we want or need to change direction. Some clients would rather have you install a turbo in their car than walk together with them. So, it requires willingness and courage from you as a therapist to teach your client to slow down. Providing an explanation of why you want to slow down can be helpful. A metaphor we often use is that of being lost in a city.

The metaphor of being lost in a new city

What is the first thing you do when you are lost in a new city? Exactly, you stop. You look around to orient yourself: where am I now? Stopping, experiencing where you are, and reorienting yourself, so that it becomes clear what the next step can be.

Slowing down a therapy session can be done in various ways. Firstly, by slowing down your own speaking pace. You can do this by simply speaking your sentences more slowly and pausing briefly after a few words. The following exercise is designed to let you experience the difference it makes.

Slowing down exercise

Read the following sentence aloud. Then, read it again, but this time, pause where the ellipses (the three dots) are placed.

1. You say that you shout at your children regularly. I can see that it is painful for you to talk about this.
2. You say… that you shout… at your children… and I see… that it is painful for you… to talk about this…

You might notice that when you speak a sentence more slowly, you not only leave more space at the ellipses but also speak the other words more slowly. This creates a slower rhythm. By slowing down, you give the client the opportunity to see what there is to see along the way. You compel the client to slow down, making it difficult for them to leave the here-and-now. This way, you create an environment where the client can look at their experience. This not only applies to the client; it also gives you more space to see what is happening, both for yourself and the client. By slowing down, you create space. Space to notice what it is. You bring the experience into the space instead of just talking about it.

In this example, you give the client the space to have experiences that arise when she acknowledges that *she* is the one who is shouting at her children. You give her the opportunity to experience what that does to her, what comes up for her when she talks about it, instead of immediately moving away from it and exploring how she can shout less.

Slowing down is a skill that you can train by simply doing it. Grant yourself the literal space to bring the pace down.

Exercise: your thoughts about slowing down

Your learning history undoubtedly tells you various things about slowing down. Take a moment to reflect on what comes up for you now. What thoughts and ideas arise when you imagine yourself slowing down a session? Write them down below ....

....

....

....

....

....

....

....

....

Slowing down is not always easy, especially with clients who tend to talk a lot. Clients who feel they must tell you everything. During an intake session, they may provide detailed accounts of their experiences, and each subsequent session starts with an extensive report of their week. When dealing with these clients, it takes courage for the therapist to slow them down. After all, their stories often revolve around there-and-then experiences, and you want to bring them into the here-and-now. An approach could be to say:

> **Example approach: establishing contact
> in the here-and-now**
>
> "You're telling me a lot, providing a lot of information; let's see what's happening here. Is that okay?
>   …This is interesting, what's happening now. Let's stay with this for a moment, okay?"

By zooming in on one aspect, you are, in a way, focusing on a few dance steps rather than the entire dance. By observing what happens around this behavior, with the client, in connection with you, you can see where it leads you and the client. It also prevents both you and the client from getting entangled in the stories the client tells. Stories that always revolve around the historical or future Self, and not about the present Self.

> **Example approach: establishing contact
> in the here-and-now**
>
> The following sentences can help you slow down and bring your client to the present moment:
>
> • "How does it feel to hear yourself telling these stories?"
> • "What is it like to experience this feeling right now?"
> • "As you look at yourself in this moment, what thoughts come to mind? What are you experiencing?"

Actively using silence

In some situations, it can be helpful to let silence fall, allowing both you and your client to notice what is happening in the here-and-now. This approach is particularly useful when either you or the client get drawn into stories. Allowing moments of silence gives you and the client the space to disentangle from these stories and focus on the experiences in the present moment. It requires willingness from both the client and the therapist to stay with the experiences in the here-and-now, so you can discover what is happening from moment-to-moment. The following sentence can be helpful in this regard:

**Example approach: establishing contact
in the here-and-now**

Shall we see if we can linger here, around this experience? Around what is
happening right now. Just try noticing what is happening.

When students practice this during our ACT training, they often give feedback
that they themselves get the thought that they are doing nothing when they allow
silences to fall. Here too, it seems that we have learned that doing something means
speaking, that we have to talk. So, it is essential to see the function of using silences
and realize that we are indeed doing something when we utilize silence.

When using silences, timing is crucial. It is not about randomly inserting a
silence. When you say something new to a client or when a client experiences
something new, you give them the time to experience and explore what is happening with a silence. Through the silence, the client doesn't need to do anything
other than notice what is happening within them. You provide the client with the
time and space to make new associations. Additionally, silences also give you the
opportunity to notice what is happening within yourself, even if it is discomfort.
Discomfort during silences can be revealing. It tells us that we have the tendency to
move away from our experience in the here-and-now. Silences can help us let go of
our stories and shift our attention to the present moment. Therefore, it is crucial to
allow yourself, as the therapist, to have moments of silence during the conversation.

I sometimes notice in myself that I am inclined to provide explanations when I
feel uncomfortable with certain silences. For example, when it is new for a client to
stay with their experience in the here-and-now, and they look at me questioningly.
I might be drawn into a story by that look – a story that tells me I am not clear, that
the client doesn't understand, that they need to understand it first to be able to do
this, that they are probably wondering if I know what I am doing, that they might
see me as an incompetent psychologist, and so on. Before I know it, I am immersed
in this story instead of maintaining contact with the client and, for instance, stating
that I can imagine it feels uncomfortable. We would like to ask you to investigate
this for yourself in a conversation with a client.

Exercise: uncomfortable silence

In a future session, notice what you do when you feel uncomfortable, and a
silence occurs. Write down below what you notice

....

....

....

....

....

....

By actively using silence, we create space to feel, space to experience what is happening in that moment. Space to let stories be stories and to connect with our experience, our heart, to notice our thoughts, let them be, and see what feelings are present, and to let those stories and thoughts settle down in our hearts.

> **Example approach: making contact in the here-and-now**
>
> When you see that your client gets pulled away from the here-and-now, you could say something like: "It's difficult to be here. Are you willing to redirect your attention back to here, to our interaction?" And once the attention is back in the here-and-now: "Where were you?"

The therapist's attitude

Of course, you can also slow down without using language, just through your demeanor as a therapist. Working in the here-and-now requires a present, active demeanor focused on the client. Sit in a comfortable position for yourself, allowing you to make optimal contact with your client. Ensure that there is nothing that can interrupt that connection. For example, I find it distracting in the interaction when I take notes. Since I've been working in a process-based way, I limit myself to jotting down factual information in the first session. In follow-up sessions, I take notes afterward so that I can be fully present with the client, with my own experiences, and with the contact between us.

> **Example approach: making contact in the here-and-now**
>
> During a conversation, I sometimes turn my head away and look at the ceiling. I am momentarily caught up in my own thoughts, and I openly

acknowledge that. For instance, I might say: "I notice that so much is happening within me, with thoughts and emotions. I'll take a moment to observe what's going on."

In this way, I show the client that it's okay to take the time to observe what's happening within oneself. It is another way of modeling behavior to be present in the here-and-now.

Other ways to create space to be in the here-and-now are slow and deep breathing, for example, when the client is feeling emotional. By doing so, you signal that it is a lot to process and that it is okay to take time to absorb it. It does not have to quickly pass because you need to move on to the next point. What next point, after all? You are where you are right now, and that is okay, and staying with that can also be very insightful.

Sometimes it is better not to work with the here-and-now

Working in the here-and-now is not always the best approach to take. In some situations, working with the here-and-now is not possible or may even lead to greater problems for the client. This has everything to do with the client's capacity to tolerate experiences. Being in the here-and-now with your experiences requires an awareness that there is an "I" and an awareness that you have experiences – an "I" with experiences. It is essential that this "I" can be seen as a safe place from which experiences can be had.

Clients who inherently struggle with this are those who are sensitive to psychosis, paranoia, delusions, and flashbacks. When you attempt to work in the here-and-now with such clients, there is a high risk that they may become more destabilized. These clients often do not have a firm and safe place from which they can experience the here-and-now. There is often no secure sense of self to experience what is happening, to be with what is unfolding in the here-and-now.

In my work with clients who have experienced severe trauma, I often use the "54321 exercise." It is an exercise that helps clients detach from their flashbacks and accompanying emotions. It involves working with the here-and-now in a different way than described in this chapter. This method helps clients who are pulled away from the present by flashbacks or reliving past experiences to redirect their attention to what is happening in the here-and-now. I teach my clients this exercise in a session by doing it together with them. The exercise goes as follows:

[Exercise] Returning to the present

The therapist starts by naming something he sees, for example, the cupboard. Then, he asks the client to do the same. The client names something he sees, for example, the blue chair. This continues until both the therapist and the client have named five things they see. Next, the therapist names something he hears, for example, the rattling of the heating system. Then, it's the client's turn again to name something he hears, for example, the ticking of the clock. This continues until both have named four things they hear. After that, the therapist names something felt on the outside of his body, for example, the pressure of the chair's armrest. Then, it is the client's turn again. Now they both name three things they feel, at the outside of the body. Finally, they can name two things they smell and one thing they taste.

In practice, I rarely include the last two senses (smell and taste). They add little to the purpose of the exercise and can make it more challenging for the client to remember. Once the exercise is complete, I ask the client what they notice. If they feel that there is more space between themselves and the experienced flashbacks/reliving, then the goal is achieved. This way, the client can gain a sense of safety when dealing with intrusive experiences.

The difference between working from your head and from your heart in the here-and-now

Throughout our lives, we have learned all sorts of things about how we should do something, how we should be, and what we should want. This applies to everyone, including our clients and ourselves as human beings and in our role as therapists. Psychologists, in general, have been taught to approach a session with their heads. We plan what we want to do before a conversation and carry out that plan, whether or not it's based on a protocol. This may not necessarily be a problem; we have been doing therapy this way for years, and many people have benefited from it. However, my experience is that a session rarely unfolds according to such a plan, which led me to believe for a long time that I was doing something wrong. This may be the case for many therapists as well.

Working from our heads can hinder working from our hearts. Consider the earlier example of my husband and our dog, Pebbels. When you follow your head, you might miss the experience that is happening at that moment (being let into a warm room) and act based on experiences in your head rather than thoughts and feelings corresponding to the present moment (the experience of being let in). The same goes for therapy. With here-and-now work, we slow down the interaction to create space between ourselves and the stories in our heads, so we can experience what is truly happening and let that experience influence our behavior. Working from the here-and-now offers an additional perspective. This perspective is not better or worse; it is merely different.

Our heart tells us how things are for us, rather than how they should be. It helps us look at our entire selves, both our pleasant and comfortable sides as well as our unpleasant and painful sides. This way, we can act based on this complete self and do what we truly want to do. By being present with the client and being in contact

with each other and with the experiences that arise, we broaden our perspective. We genuinely connect with ourselves, the client, and everything that arises. Clients often tell us that they feel seen by us and that they feel we truly understand them. What they experience is that, through working with the here-and-now, we work from our hearts, as human beings with human beings. It becomes possible to look at everything, both experiences from the head and those from the heart.

Working with the here-and-now also helps us recognize when we are pulled away from our hearts. It helps us teach the client to see in which situations they are pushed in a direction other than where they truly want to go. The therapist's task is to recognize and name this movement. For example, when you see that the client is moved, experiencing an emotion, and quickly starts talking, you could say:

Example approach: contacting the here-and-now

"May I interrupt you? You just started talking, but I believe something significant just happened. Is it okay to take a look at that?"

Or sometimes even more concise: "May I ask you to stop talking for a moment. Is it okay to stay with this experience, with what is happening now?"

Beginning to talk when experiencing an emotion is not the only signal that a client is pulled away from their experience and into their head. When a client suddenly switches to another topic, changes their tone, shifts in their seat, or looks away, these can all be behavioral signals that the client is moving away from their experience in the here-and-now.

By naming these changes in behavior as a therapist, you show the client that they are having an experience and are apparently choosing to move away from it. By making this visible, naming it, and then suggesting alternative behavior, such as stopping talking and experiencing what they feel, you create a context in which the client can exhibit different behavior.

We can teach this to the client only when we ourselves can be in the here-and-now, when we are willing to work from our hearts. This means that as therapists, we must be willing to let go of protocols, abandon predetermined plans, and be willing to work from our experience, from our compassionate contact with ourselves and with our client. This is working from your heart.

Behavior is only directly influenced from the here-and-now

We often talk about things we would have liked to do differently or want to do in the future. However, we cannot change our behavior from there-and-then. The past has happened; it is over. It went as it did. We can only make representations of the future. But even in the present, we can do nothing about it. We can visualize where we want to go, but we can only set our feet in that direction from the here-and-now.

Working from the here-and-now is essential because it allows us much more influence to potentially change our client's behavior. A good example of this is the example of going to the gym. At night, when I lie in bed, I often think: tomorrow I will go to the gym. I am sure I will do it. However, in the here-and-now of the next day, there is always something that prevents me from going. In our thoughts, we can plan to do something, but we can only move our feet and take actual steps in the here-and-now.

As therapists, we often work the same way. We talk about behavior as it is and as it should be. We ask the client to do things differently in the weeks between therapy sessions. Some clients do a lot of work between sessions; others do not. That is not good or bad; it is a context in which you, as the therapist, have little or no influence. A context where you have no control over what happens, which steps the client takes, and which direction the dance is going. It is like telling the client what a new dance looks like and asking them to practice it at home without rehearsing these steps together and without being able to give them direct feedback.

With here-and-now work, you practice the steps in the session. Together with your client, you experience what it is like to take these new steps so that the client can create new dances. Here you can exert influence because the interaction between you and the client is in the here-and-now. Here you can teach the client new behavior. To experience this yourself, you can do the following exercise:

Time machine metaphor exercise

The way our brain functions is a bit like a time machine. It is as if we can jump to the past and the future whenever we want. We jump to the past, and our thoughts bring us back to the experiences and emotions of that time, far back. We can see, hear, smell... how it was, and it feels like we are back there. Now, close your eyes and jump to a past experience. What do you see, hear, feel, and think? Notice how what you experienced there, you experience as here-and-now.

We can also jump forward. Our thoughts take us to what we desire, what we have been seeking for a long time, and the experiences and emotions from that time in the future are ours to feel. Now, close your eyes and jump to a projected experience in the future. What do you see, hear, feel, and think? What you will experience there, you experience as here-and-now.

Now, really open your eyes and experience the present moment. Be here-and-now. What you hear, see, smell, think, feel...

Did you notice a difference between being in the past, being in the future, and being here? From which position can you genuinely make a difference, use your hands and feet? (Harris, 2009)

Working from the here-and-now is essential because it allows us much more influence to potentially change our client's behavior.

Case Margaret: part 2

At the beginning of therapy, Margaret struggled to stay in the here-and-now. She was often caught up in 'there-and-then' thinking, saying that her life would be better if she were free from her symptoms. To initiate here-and-now work, I started by slowing down the pace of my speech. I would say things like, "I understand that you're in a lot of pain" or "I can imagine how difficult it is for you to have so many symptoms." In the first two sessions, Margaret responded immediately, answering quickly with statements like, "Yes, it definitely is." She would then continue to talk about all the things she could no longer do. By using shorter sentences like, "Pff, [sighing deeply] … this is painful," and then saying, "Take a moment to notice what you're experiencing right now," I gradually brought Margaret into the here-and-now.

During the third session, Margaret fell silent for the first time and checked in with what she was experiencing at that moment. It lasted only a few seconds before she said, "I just want to feel better." I could respond by saying something like, "Yes… this is what's happening. It's difficult for you to stay with what's happening right now, and that's okay." I acknowledged that Margaret was practicing moving back and forth between the here-and-now at her own pace. It is essential to do this slowly over several sessions instead of just giving Margaret mindfulness exercises. She had undoubtedly done those exercises before, but her goal was always to get rid of her symptoms as quickly as possible. After about six sessions, there was sadness. Margaret felt tears streaming down her face and wiped them away vigorously, saying, "Yeah, this is not what I signed up for." After a moment of silence, I responded by saying, "Yes… this is difficult… to feel." Margaret also remained silent and nodded.

This slow pattern of moving back and forth between bringing attention to the here-and-now and following Margaret's stories allowed her to get to know the here-and-now and gain trust to stay there longer. It also gave Margaret a sense of control. The freedom to leave the here-and-now when she needed to. By experiencing this sense of control, Margaret became better at going to the here-and-now and staying there even outside of therapy sessions.

Margaret can now readily connect with her pain and sadness, allowing her to explore them, and let them be a part of her life. In that way, Margaret can see herself completely and, from there, decide what she wants to do.

Summary and conclusion

Working in the here-and-now is often associated with mindfulness exercises. However, in this chapter, we have explained that here-and-now work goes beyond that. Working in the here-and-now is about being present, fully in touch with yourself, with your client, and with whatever is happening between you, moment-by-moment. What is happening can be seen as a dance, and through here-and-now work, we gain more insight into the steps that make up this dance, how we experience these steps, and where they lead.

Nevertheless, it is not easy to work in the here-and-now. We often have not learned to be with our experiences in the here-and-now and instead prefer "there-and-then" thinking. As therapists, we also tend to focus on positive outcomes, often associated with being good practitioners. Moreover, language can easily pull us out of our experiences and into our thoughts, often without us realizing it. Finally, our experiences in the here-and-now are often too painful, causing us to naturally retreat rather than stay with them.

We have shown how you can learn to work in the here-and-now. By slowing down the pace of a session, creating space for the experience through the use of functional silence, and adopting an accepting attitude. Working in the here-and-now is not always suitable, especially for clients who cannot experience a safe place within themselves. These are clients who often have psychotic or paranoid experiences or who have severe flashbacks.

Working in the here-and-now enables us to let go of working mainly from our heads and work more from our hearts. To work from our direct experience in contact with others, from person to person. This broader perspective allows us to not only direct our lives from our heads but also from our hearts. Lastly, we have emphasized that as a therapist, you have the most influence on behavioral change in direct interaction with your client, and that is in the here-and-now.

Reference

Harris, R. (2009). *ACT made simple: An easy-to-read primer on acceptance and commitment therapy*. Oakland: New Harbinger Publications.

Chapter 6

Acceptance and willingness to embrace discomfort

Marjolein Vleugel

In this chapter, I will demonstrate how acceptance and willingness can assist both the therapist and the client in coping with their psychological pain. Humans have a natural tendency to avoid pain as well as situations that might trigger it. This tendency is often referred to as experiential avoidance. Evolutionarily, this inclination to distance oneself from physical pain is a logical solution. When your house is on fire, it is entirely rational to try to get out of the house as quickly as possible. However, we often approach psychological pain in a similar manner. In this chapter, I will discuss why this might not always be the best strategy to deal with such pain and explore how acceptance and willingness offer an alternative to experiential avoidance.

Firstly, I will begin the chapter by explaining what is meant by acceptance. Acceptance involves learning to (willingly) observe and acknowledge pain within us and in our lives. It also involves actively inviting the dark and painful aspects of ourselves and/or our lives so that we can experience them. This process of observing, acknowledging, and inviting pain can be a significant challenge, both for the client and the therapist. Therefore, it is essential that the therapist has also experienced what it is like to avoid their own pain and, therefore, what it is like to choose to move toward it. As such, I will explore how to enhance willingness in both the client and in oneself.

Working with acceptance and willingness is an ongoing process. It is not something that can be achieved and never lost again. At times, we may be more willing and, at other times, less willing to embrace all our experiences in life.

Sophie: part 1 of case study

Sophie, 38 years old, seeks help from a therapist regarding concerns around her relationship with her daughter. Her daughter does not listen to her, and Sophie does not have this problem with her two younger children. Frequent arguments occur, driving Sophie to despair, and she finds herself frequently shouting at the children. Sophie is at her wit's end, and motherhood has not turned out as she had imagined. She cannot comprehend what is wrong with her daughter and has already sought

DOI: 10.4324/9781032699691-7

help for her daughter from a child psychologist. She hopes to receive guidance from me on how to handle her daughter differently so that things can improve at home.

From the initial information provided by Sophie, it becomes evident that she has a certain idea of what motherhood should be like, how her behavior as a mother should be, and how her children should behave. However, the reality is different, and this discrepancy is causing problems. When ideas about how the world should be significantly differ from the reality, working with acceptance and willingness becomes crucial.

From acceptance to willingness

When clients come to us for therapy, they often hear that they should simply "accept" things. This can refer to various aspects, such as dealing with loss, self-perception, unpleasant experiences like pain, or emotions like fear, sadness, or irritability. We are discussing the psychological and sometimes physical pain experienced by the client. However, "just accepting it" is easier said than done. What does acceptance actually mean? And what exactly is there to accept?

Acceptance is a crucial component of acceptance and commitment therapy (ACT). However, both our clients and us as therapists have varying ideas about the meaning of the word "acceptance." When we ask our students, for instance, what acceptance means to them, we receive diverse responses. They define acceptance as "embracing what you feel," "tolerating," "being okay with what is happening or has happened," or "finding peace with what you have experienced," among other interpretations.

When we say that we have accepted something, it often implies that we are no longer bothered by that "something." In our view, acceptance is not about no longer being affected by something. Instead, acceptance is about seeing, acknowledging, and experiencing what is present within you and your life, even if it is painful, difficult, or unpleasant. This seeing, acknowledging, and experiencing can only occur when you are willing to look at that "something," regardless of what it may be. Therefore, the way we approach acceptance is through willingness. When we talk about acceptance, the question is whether you are willing to open your eyes. With your eyes open, you can see what is there, right now, in your life. Are you willing to acknowledge what is happening now? Willingness involves shining a light on the darker aspects of yourself. This is necessary to see what you are doing. Being willing to actively embrace this darkness into your life allows you to see, acknowledge, and experience your complete self, which in turn enables you to act from this place.

Allowing the dark aspects of yourself

It is a very natural response to move away from something painful. Think again about the example of the burning house. We evacuate the house, move away, leave the danger, and avoid the pain. It becomes more challenging when the fire is not in our house but within ourselves. When the pain is something within us, and if we walk away, we simply carry the pain with us.

I like to use the metaphor of Yin and Yang in my sessions.

The Yin and Yang metaphor

Yin represents the black part and symbolizes our dark and negative aspects. Yang, on the other hand, represents the white part and symbolizes our light and positive aspects. Yin and yang together form a whole. We are yin *and* yang. Whether we want to acknowledge it or not, we are never solely yin or solely yang. Avoiding our painful experiences is similar to excluding either yin (black) or yang (white). However, we often prefer to exclude the darker aspects of ourselves rather than the lighter ones. When you exclude a part of yourself, it doesn't mean that it disappears and no longer influences your actions. After all, it is a part of you. By cultivating willingness, being open to examining Yin (black) as well as Yang (white), you can see what else belongs to you. It allows you to observe what drives your behavior in addition to yang (white). This way, you get a more complete picture of yourself – a picture of how and who you are, rather than just a certain limited version of yourself, for example, solely yang (white).

Like everyone else, I know that I can be unkind at times, that I may burden others, cause them sadness, and that I make mistakes. I experience fear and anger too. Knowing all this doesn't necessarily mean that I am okay with it. I would prefer not to exhibit or be any of those things. Just like any other human being, I am inclined to focus on how I can behave better – how I can be kinder, cause less trouble for my loved ones, prevent causing pain and sorrow to them and others, and avoid making mistakes.

That seems logical, right? After all, who wouldn't want to constantly display the best version of themselves? The tricky part is that, as humans, we are not always the best version of ourselves, and we don't always feel our best, which means we cannot always present the best version of ourselves. We are, after all, yin and yang.

The point here is not about what we want; it is about the fact that we are all humans and sometimes, by nature, display unkind or unpleasant behavior or have negative thoughts. However, trying to look away from our dark side and expand our lighter side to eliminate the dark side doesn't work. We remain yin and yang, and we will never become purely yang (white). In fact, it is impossible to ever be completely yin (black) or yang (white). We can't help but accept this fact – accepting that we are humans. My efforts to be as much yang (white) as possible may lead me to perfect my yang, but it doesn't mean that I lose my yin (black) in the process. It is a bit like spending all my time at the gym to maximize my left side and ignoring my right side. A perfectly trained left side does not make a perfect body. Focusing solely on training the left side does not eliminate the limitations of my right side, no matter how much time and effort I put into it. For my entire body to function better, I need to see and acknowledge that there is also a right side. A right side that also contributes to how my body functions. I can better control my behavior when I am willing to look at all aspects of it – both the pleasant, positive sides and the painful and unpleasant experiences. We invite you to take a look at your own yin and yang as well.

Exercise: Yin and Yang sides of you

Write down your dark and painful aspects that you would rather not have. These can be characteristics or experiences that you possess or have had and would prefer not to have or be associated with.

....

....

....

....

....

....

....

....

....

....

....

....

It is necessary to have the willingness to look at your dark and often painful sides and acknowledge their existence in order to understand how these aspects influence your behavior. When you cannot see something, you have no idea how it affects your behavior. Pretending it is not there is like a little child covering their eyes and thinking they are invisible to others. Acting as if your dark and painful side does not exist does not make it disappear or stop influencing your actions.

Welcoming and including experiences

Once we are willing to look at what we find difficult or unpleasant, the next step is to openly invite in these experiences. The goal is not to be free from pain; the goal is to be able to do what you truly want to do, even with your pain.

A metaphor that fits well here is the "uninvited guest" (Hayes et al., 1999).

The metaphor of the uninvited guest

You are hosting a party and have invited everyone except that one person who always looks a bit disheveled, has an unpleasant odor, and behaves differently from others. The party is lively and in full swing, and you are having a great time with your guests. Suddenly, you see someone walking by the windows outside, peering inside. You go to see who it is, and, to your dismay, it's that uninvited person. You decide to close the curtains and turn back to your guests, hoping they haven't noticed anything. Then, you hear a knock on the door. You open it and find that it's the uninvited guest again. You ask him to leave and quickly close the door, looking at your guests to see if they've noticed anything. You join them again, hoping he has finally left and won't bother you anymore. But then, you hear the doorbell ring. You decide to ignore it, but unfortunately, it keeps ringing. Everyone hears the long, insistent sound, and you can no longer pretend not to hear it. You open the door and almost shout at the person to leave. You decide to sit by the door so that he cannot enter unnoticed. After a while, you feel miserable. You hear your guests laughing while you are sitting far away from everyone, barricading the door to prevent the uninvited guest from coming in. You decide to rejoin your guests because you enjoy being with them, and you realize you prefer that over barricading the door all the time to keep the uninvited guest out. You have fun with your guests and notice that the uninvited guest has found a way to enter. You may feel disappointed and tense, realizing that pretending he's not there doesn't work. Perhaps you also notice that even with the uninvited guest at the party, you can still enjoy conversations with your guests. Of course, you would prefer him not to be at your party, but at least you are no longer stuck by the door, away from your own party. The party goes on, and you notice that the uninvited guest no longer demands your attention all the time. He still looks disheveled, still smells unpleasant, and still behaves differently from the others, but he seems much calmer. You also see him making some jokes with some of your friends.

This metaphor illustrates that willingness is about including all feelings, thoughts, and experiences, both unpleasant and pleasant, not in a way of preparing for a battle by saying, "Bring it on, I can handle you," but instead, welcoming all experiences and being ready to embrace them by saying, "I see you, you are a part of me," and extending welcome to them.

When you allow the uninvited guest to enter, it does not mean that suddenly he starts smelling good. He still stinks, and his behavior is still odd. However, by letting this smelly, peculiar guest in, it creates space for you to mingle with the other guests. You no longer have to keep an eye on the door or be on guard that the uninvited guest might sneak in unnoticed because he is already there.

Actively opening yourself to what is painful for you is like inviting an uninvited guest. Being willing to experience this pain allows you to function as a complete and whole human being (yin and yang) instead of just a part of yourself (e.g., only yang). Sometimes, we need the help of another person to open the door for the uninvited guests. It is not easy to open that door when everything inside you almost screams to keep it closed. Someone else can assist you in taking that courageous step. Someone who is willing to look with you at your yin (black) – your dark, painful aspects – to examine and experience them. So that you can be your complete self again, instead of a "perfect" but half version of yourself.

Acceptance and willingness in both the client and therapist

When we ask our clients to look at their pain and open the door, we are asking a lot of them. It is important for us, as therapists, to have experienced how it is to work with willingness, so we can understand what we are asking from our clients. First and foremost, to have personally experienced how challenging it can be to face and embrace what is painful and difficult in life. Secondly, to be fully present with ourselves as therapists and in the relationship with our clients, opening to both our strengths and vulnerabilities. Moreover, it helps us to be an example for our clients in working with willingness.

Acceptance does not mean that you never feel insecure as a therapist. It is about being willing to experience insecurity and realizing that you are still okay as a person and as a therapist. By increasing your willingness, you can learn to examine your insecurities and see how they influence your behavior, so you can gain more control over your actions instead of letting insecurities control you.

Being willing to be where you are

Many people strive to become a better version of themselves, essentially wanting to be someone else than who they are. I am certainly no exception to this. In fact, I can honestly say it is one of my biggest struggles. Always wanting to know more, achieve better results, feel better, be more yang (white) than yin (black). On the outside, it may look mostly positive. People see someone who is cheerful and kind, works hard, and is knowledgeable. However, inside, a struggle arises – the belief that I should be different from who I am, always happy and kind, working even harder, knowing even more, and becoming a better therapist than I am. This battle between the reality of who I am and how I think I should be, costs me energy.

If I keep fighting this battle, I eventually become exhausted because I can never be endlessly happier, kinder, work harder, or know more. There is no end to it. Acceptance involves asking: Am I willing to know what I know now? Am I willing to be who I am now, as a person and as a therapist?

Ironically, by repeatedly increasing my willingness to look at myself as a whole, acknowledging that I am both yin and yang, it creates more space. A sense of relief arises because I've let go of the struggle to be something other than who I am, to experience something other than what I'm experiencing. I must admit that it does not happen automatically and is not always easy. It is sad to see that I hurt others at times because I am not always kind and cheerful. It is disheartening to admit that I make mistakes and don't always have all the answers. At the same time, I experience space and a weight lifted off my shoulders. A complete realization that I am who I am, yin and yang, and that is okay. I do not have to be anything other than who I am, as a person and as a therapist.

Let's see if you can experience this for yourself with the following exercise.

Exercise: willingness move

Think of something that is difficult for you. For example, something you struggle with in your work or personal life, like applying something new in a therapy session, addressing a colleague, setting boundaries with your children, or ending a relationship. Choose something that is challenging for you. Once you have it in mind, I want to ask you the following: If you want to move toward acceptance, what do you need to be willing to face? Notice how this feels for you and write it down...

....

....

....

....

....

....

....

....

....

....

....

....

Being willing to let the client be where they are

As humans and therapists, we never reach a point where we know everything. There's always room to learn. I vividly remember sitting at the table with my former supervisor, who was twice my age when I was 21. I looked up to him because he knew so much. I told him that I couldn't wait to be his age so that I would know exactly what to do with my clients. He burst out laughing, and I now understand why.

Process-based ACT, like other behavioral therapies, focuses on behavioral change. However, that does not mean that as a therapist, you have complete control over the pace and form of this change. As you have read in the previous chapter, we can only influence the client's behavior in the here and now. As therapists, we follow the client where they are, and it is our task to create a context in which the client can learn new behavior. Whether they do it, when they do it, and how they do it is the client's responsibility. What it requires from us as therapists is a willingness to let the client walk their path, at their own pace and in their own way.

It can emotionally demand a lot from clients to confront difficult issues. As therapists, we must not forget that we are not the ones in the client's shoes. The client is responsible for their behavior, and thus they are the ones who must bear the consequences of any behavioral changes. It is up to us, as therapists, to accept that the client does this at their own pace and in their own way. This requires the therapist's acceptance and willingness to follow the client in this process.

That can be quite challenging. In both the societal context and from the client's side, there are often high expectations from us as healthcare providers. The idea prevails that the therapist knows what the client should do to feel better and that he knows which "buttons" should be pressed in order to quickly and without complications achieve a good end result. It also seems to be the expectation that the client will do exactly what is necessary to achieve this result without straying. For example, wanting the client to sleep better than they currently do or expecting the client to work more hours than they can handle. The reality is usually much more complex. We often get pulled into the narrative that we need to achieve results faster with our clients. We then tend to pull the client to a point at which we believe they should be, or wish they already were.

But who are we to determine that a client must confront their dark sides? We can only show the consequences of not facing them. The client is and remains the one who chooses whether or not to do this and to live with the consequences of their choices. They are responsible for their behavior and no one else. The client is a free person, free to choose. It is your task to show that there are multiple options when the client is willing to explore multiple options. The question for you is: Are you willing to allow all that freedom for your client?

The client sets the pace

When clients first come to your office, they share a lot about themselves, their experiences, and what they do or do not do. From your perspective as a therapist, you establish connections between what the client has experienced and their behavior. You are trained to see these connections. However, the client has often never looked at their behavior and learning history in this way before.

For example, a client may express feeling very down and unhappy but claim not to know why. After all, they have everything in their life – a good job, a beautiful and healthy family, and enough money in the bank to buy whatever they want. It becomes apparent to the therapist that the client has mainly lived according to what they thought they should do, rather than doing what they truly wanted to do. The realization that they are now unhappy because they didn't do what they wanted to do can be a painful one for the client.

The therapist helps the client make these painful connections visible so that the client can acknowledge that this is about their life and about their pain. When the client sees and acknowledges their pain, they can work on being willing to actively embrace this pain in their life. The willingness to see, acknowledge, and experience pain varies from one client to another. It requires patience from the therapist to follow the client's pace in this process. It is only when the client indicates they are willing to take a step, that we should go along with them. It is as if we ask the client to step into an ice bath. We do not want to push the client underwater because we think it might be good for them. Instead, we guide the client step by step into the bath when they are ready, at their pace. After all, they are the ones getting into the bath.

I must admit that I am not always patient. Instead of being patient and following the client's pace and behavior, I take action. I start working hard, for example, by giving more explanations or by telling the client how to get into the ice bath in the best way. The problem is that giving explanations feels good. After all, I don't have to experience my impatience. The client often perceives it as something positive as well because they don't have to face their pain either. The unfortunate part is that, although this may feel good for both the therapist and the client, no progress is made in the direction of the client's willingness to look at their painful and difficult aspects.

It is up to the therapist to show the client what they see, to create the context so that the client can establish conclusions on their own. Making these conclusions for the client, imposing them on them, is futile. These conclusions may undoubtedly reach the client's mind, but there is a high chance that they will remain there and not be integrated into their experience, into their heart.

The client makes their own choices

The fundamental principle in therapy is that the client is responsible for their behavior. They determine what they do or do not do. After all, they are the ones who must bear the consequences of their actions. While this may sound simple and logical, therapists often find it challenging to accept. I, too, sometimes think, "Just do it." However, there is a reason why someone may not be doing or be able to do something yet. It is up to us to make the client aware of the steps they are taking and the consequences that result from their behavior. It is up to us to accept whether the client is willing or unwilling to look at these aspects and whether they will or will not do something differently.

We can suggest, for instance, that a client should take more time for themselves. However, we are not the ones who can action that. We are not the ones who have to bear the consequences of that new behavior, whatever those consequences may be. The client must be willing to do so, often not knowing what the consequences of this new behavior might be (yet). Only when the client is willing to bear all the consequences, whether they are easy, challenging, or painful, can they take responsibility for their behavior.

This is also the goal of process-based ACT: to show the client that they are free to choose. When the therapist makes the choice, we are depriving them of that freedom. Yes, sometimes it is hard for us as therapists when the client chooses (still) to remain in a painful or difficult situation. That is something the therapist has to accept.

Placing this responsibility on the client is a common thread in process-based work. After all, we do not have a predefined outcome in terms of, for example, experiencing less anxiety or improving mood (as in more traditional therapies). The outcome is that the client learns to see what they are doing, why they are doing it, and is willing to take other steps to move in a direction they truly want to go.

What does working with acceptance and willingness look like?

Practicing willingness

Willingness is a skill that can be trained. An initial introduction to willingness is covered in the following exercise:

Exercise willingness and rules

Write down ten rules that you believe a therapist should follow:

1. ....
2. ....
3. ....
4. ....
5. ....
6. ....
7. ....
8. ....
9. ....

10. ....

Now, I invite you to choose one rule that you will break in the coming week. Which one would that be?

....

What do you experience now, thinking about breaking that rule? Do you feel discomfort or something else? The question is: are you willing to experience what it's like to break this rule, to behave differently than you are used to? Are you willing to have those experiences, regardless of the consequences?

Keep track of your experiences in the time leading up to breaking the rule, during the process of breaking the rule, and afterward.

This exercise is a simple intervention to introduce yourself and your clients to willingness. A willingness to step out of your comfort zone. When we stay within our comfort zone, we narrow our lives due to a need for safety. Consequently, we may miss opportunities outside that comfort zone, which could enrich our lives. By doing things differently than we are used to, we may gain new experiences.

Actively engaging with willingness

To illustrate to clients that we tend to confine ourselves to a comfort zone, doing what we've always done (even if it may no longer be effective), we use the

---

The metaphor of the radio knobs (and the wrench) (Hayes et al., 1999)

Imagine we have a radio here with two sliding knobs, like the balance and volume knobs. One knob is the volume knob that can go louder and softer [move your hand up and down], and the other knob is the balance knob. Let's call one of them "anxiety" [move your hand up and down as if on a numerical scale]. It can range from 0 to 10. You came here because it's too high [move your hand from bottom to top]. You want to bring it down, and you want me, your therapist, to help you with that. In other words, you've tried to slide this control down the scale, but it hasn't worked [the therapist can use the other hand to unsuccessfully pull down the "anxiety" hand].

However, there is another scale we call "willingness." It represents how open you are to experiencing your own feelings as they are, without trying to manipulate, avoid, change, or escape them, etc. This scale also ranges from 0 to 10.

What we do in therapy is make this scale more visible to you. It is also the most crucial of the two because this is the scale that makes a difference, and it's the only scale you can control.

When "anxiety" is at 10, and you try hard to control it, make it decrease or disappear, you are not willing to feel that anxiety. In other words, the willingness scale is at 0 at that moment. And honestly, that's a terrible combination.

It's like a wrench. When you set the wrench in one direction, no matter how hard you turn the handle, it can only tighten the bolt. The same goes for you. When anxiety is high, and willingness is low, the bolt is tightly screwed, and anxiety cannot decrease. If you are not willing to experience anxiety, anxiety becomes something to worry about. When anxiety is high, and willingness decreases, it's like anxiety gets stuck. You turn the wrench, and no matter what you do, it tightens the bolt even more.

So what we need to do in this therapy is shift our focus from the anxiety scale to the willingness scale. You've been trying to control anxiety for a long time, and it just doesn't work. It's not that you're not working hard enough or not smart enough; focusing on and trying to control your anxiety simply doesn't work. Instead, we direct our attention to the willingness scale.

Unlike the anxiety scale, which you can't move up and down freely, the willingness scale is a knob that you can set and slide at will. When you came in here, your willingness scale was set low. What we need to do is get it to a high level. If you do that, if you set your willingness high, I can already predict what will happen with anxiety.

When you stop trying to control your anxiety, when you set your willingness scale high, your anxiety will be low … [pause] or … it will be high. One of the two, for sure. And if it's low, it will stay low until it's not low anymore, Then it will be low again… I'm not fooling you here.

There's just no other way to explain how willingness works, how it feels to have the willingness scale set high. But I can say one thing for sure, and you've experienced it yourself too. If you want to be absolutely sure where the anxiety scale will be, there's something you can do. Simply set the willingness scale very, very low, and sooner or later, when anxiety starts, the wrench will tighten the bolt completely, and you'll have a lot of anxiety. It will be very predictable. All this effort in order to lower anxiety, but it never works. However, if you slide the willingness scale up, anxiety is free to move. Sometimes it will be low, and sometimes it will be high, and in both cases, you stay away from a useless and unpleasant struggle that can only lead in one direction.

following metaphor. In this example, we use 'fear' as the thing the client avoids, but you can replace it with whatever is applicable to you or your client.

With this metaphor, you pave the way to work with willingness. The client can learn to notice when their willingness scale is low and when they raise it.

When the willingness scale goes up, and anxiety can move back and forth, the client may become capable of looking at anxiety. They can explore what the anxiety is about and why it might be present. Through this process, they can experience that anxiety is not something to fear. By increasing their willingness, they can bring aspects of their life into visibility and see how they influence their lives. The client learns to recognize how anxiety has been directing their life. By being willing to have anxiety in their life, they can regain control and steer their life instead of being controlled by anxiety.

I vividly remember a time when I had fixed my volume knob during a training session. I was stuck in the story that I was doing terribly and not doing anything right. I felt extremely stressed, couldn't eat anything during the lunch break, and even considered quitting the course at that moment. During a break, I allowed myself to sit with this feeling, and as a result, I started crying intensely. I was willing to feel what I felt – the stress, tension, and pain in my stomach. I noticed that I wanted to know everything already and that I should be doing much better than I perceived. Then a thought occurred to me: "Okay, Marjolein, if you're such a lousy trainer, are you willing to let this be the worst course you've ever taught? If not, then cancel everything and ask a colleague to finish this training." I felt myself becoming calmer, and I realized that I was willing to do this, so I completed the course. The question is, what are you willing to face? What is present now, and are you willing to experience it? And if it is there, what calls for willingness?

However, it is not easy and automatic to raise the willingness knob. This is only possible from a kind of safe place within yourself. A place from which it is okay, and you feel safe to look at and experience painful matters. We refer to this as "self-as-context," which we will discuss more in the next chapter.

What is important to know for now is that clients who come to therapy may not always have such a place, know of it, or be in that place. They are consumed by their symptoms and painful issues, and they may not be able to look at those matters from that internal standpoint. Before we ask our clients to increase their willingness, they must first experience a place within themselves from which they can observe and experience those issues.

Learning to stay with the pain

One way to increase willingness in your client is demonstrated in the following transcript. This exercise shows how you can enable your client to look at and experience their feelings together with you.

Transcript: increasing willingness

[Therapist and client conversation]
Therapist: Alright, shall we explore how willingness might look like?
Client: Sure, what should I do?

Therapist: Earlier, you mentioned your family. What do you experience when you talk about them?

Client: I notice a surge of frustration.

Therapist: Okay, let's take a step back and observe this frustration from a distance. What do you feel in your body when you do that?

Client: I feel pain in my stomach.

Therapist: Make contact with that pain in your stomach. Imagine you can see the pain, what shape or color does it have?

Client: It's hard, dark, and bleak.

Therapist: What does that pain tell you? What comes to mind when you focus on that pain in your stomach?

Client: I'm not quite sure what you mean?

Therapist: You don't have to do anything else but notice the pain in your stomach. Keep your attention there and simply observe what arises.

Client: Anger. I notice that I feel angry.

Therapist: Lean back in your chair, take a breath. [The therapist takes an audible breath.] Now, see if you're willing to let the pain, this anger, come forth in this room, where we are now, sitting in this chair.

Client: I feel the pain; it's like my stomach is upset, and it will never settle down. It hurts. Therapist: [in a calm and soothing tone] Here we sit, together with your pain… Me here with you… You on your chair… Willing to feel your pain, in your stomach… You are here … and here is your pain. Breathe calmly, feel the pain in your stomach… Be willing to sit with your pain. Notice what happens.

In this transcript, the client is guided to be present to something painful in their life. They feel it in their stomach, and the therapist takes all the time to stay there with them. By staying with the pain, the client can have new experiences. They can realize that they are capable of staying with the pain. Sometimes, this might only be for a short while, and then it is up to the therapist to reinforce this new behavior, no matter how brief, by acknowledging how courageous it is for the client to welcome, and be willing to experience this pain.

This process helps the client to experience that they have a choice. Going toward the pain becomes an option alongside avoiding the pain. Nobody else but the client can determine whether they should move toward their pain or not. Through this work, we offer an alternative. The client learns that they are also capable of moving toward their pain, so they can choose to do so when it works better for them than avoidance. This way, the client can experience having more control over their life. Through this new behavior, they can decide to move toward the pain themselves, instead of the pain pushing them automatically in the direction of avoidance.

What if willingness is low?

Low willingness in the therapist

Being willing as a therapist to be where you are also means being willing to allow all experiences to be present in a session, both yours and your client's experiences. This can be emotionally demanding for you as a therapist. Being present with your client's painful and difficult experiences can take an emotional toll. We constantly find ourselves close to another person's suffering, and it can leave us affected. Sometimes, we might be less willing to fully allow all experiences to be present.

Signs of low willingness in a therapist can include:

- Emotional detachment
- Telling the client what they should do
- Providing explanations or analyzing what is happening
- Trying to rescue the client from their negative feelings

Perhaps you tend to provide explanations when your willingness is low, or you try to come up with solutions. Maybe you recognize yourself in all the mentioned examples. We invite you to do the following exercise during your upcoming sessions:

Exercise: low willingness

Notice what you do when your willingness is low in your next sessions. Record what you observe ....

....

....

....

I frequently notice that my willingness is low, especially when I have many clients in a day or when several clients are experiencing significant pain. I find it more challenging to be fully present in the contact, and I realize that I am more inclined to provide explanations about what I perceive is going on or what should happen. I observe these patterns, and if possible, I adjust my schedule accordingly. I learn to be compassionate with myself by acknowledging that I am also human. This means that I am willing to accept that I am not always willing.

By being aware of our own willingness and recognizing when it is low, we can work toward improving our presence and responsiveness as therapists. Embracing our own limitations and taking care of ourselves emotionally will allow us to be more effective and empathetic in our therapeutic work.

Low willingness in the client

It is possible that your client chooses to keep their willingness low. Often, the client hopes that there is another, easier way to live fully from a place of authenticity. However, there is no other way than through acceptance and willingness. We cannot live fully with our hands covering our eyes. We cannot pretend that our body consists only of the left side while ignoring the right side. As a therapist, you cannot push the willingness button up for your client; they must do it themselves.

It is important to realize that removing our hands from our eyes is difficult because we are so accustomed to keeping them there, even though we know it doesn't work. For instance, a client of mine had already undergone various treatments to overcome his flashbacks, but none of them had worked. In our sessions, we worked on increasing acceptance and willingness to let these flashbacks be part of his life without trying to change or get rid of them. The client often admitted that he secretly hoped the flashbacks would disappear.

When the client expressed this desire, I acknowledged that it is a logical wish. For example, I might say, "I understand that you want to get rid of these flashbacks, and yet, they are here now, in your life." By acknowledging where the client currently stands, where he is willing to look at right now, you can add something. In this case, I added, "they are here now, in your life." This created an opportunity for the client to increase his willingness. When he did so, he might sigh, become quiet, and experience sadness. Sometimes, this happened; other times, it did not. On those occasions, the client became angry and talked about why he thought he had these symptoms.

The therapist creates a context in which it is possible for the client to increase their willingness. We can slow down the pace, take smaller steps. Whether the client increases their willingness or not is entirely their choice each time. In my experience, almost all clients appreciate this freedom of choice. Their struggle to change their behavior is acknowledged, and they are given the opportunity to do so at their own pace.

We are never done with acceptance and willingness

In this chapter, you have learned that acceptance is about being willing to see pain, acknowledging its existence, seeing it in yourself, and actively allowing it to be part of your life. Over and over again, whenever pain emerges, being willing to see it, acknowledge it, and allow it in.

Specific pain related to a particular event may become less burdensome over time. For example, losing a loved one. After a while, you may not cry every day anymore. However, the pain, the sorrow, can suddenly resurface. You hear a song on the radio that reminds you of the person you lost. You miss them, and you notice that you feel sad. Even after 30 years, the pain and sorrow can return.

A few years ago, I experienced something distressing. I knew immediately that I needed time and space to fully experience all the emotions surrounding this event. I cleared my schedule, took time off work, and sought support. In short, I saw my pain, acknowledged that it was there in my life, and was willing to experience it … for a week. Because after a week, I felt that I had cried enough, and it was time to get back to work. I resumed work and noticed that I couldn't concentrate, and feelings of grief still overwhelmed me regularly. I became angry and indignant, wondering why I was still struggling with this. Hadn't I accepted it? Wasn't

Exercise: willingness to experience

Take a moment to think about this: What if, to live your life the way you truly want to live it, you had to be willing to feel the most painful emotions in your life? Reflect on this. If this is the price you need to pay for a healthy or fulfilling life, are you willing to do it? What comes to mind when you think about it?

....

....

....

....

....

....

....

I willing to experience all those intense emotions? Apparently, there was more to feel, to experience. Acknowledging this and being willing once again to have these difficult experiences required much more effort than in the first week.

We have no control over which pain we encounter in our lives, when it will appear, and to what extent it will affect us. What we do have control over is our willingness scale. Can we push it up when needed, even when we tell ourselves that we are done with it?

The question of acceptance and willingness is always present. When we get stuck, when we encounter pain in our lives, the questions will always be: "What is the pain?" and "Am I willing to experience it?" Then we can choose whether to push up our willingness scale.

Acceptance and willingness are not just concepts. They are not feelings, and certainly not strategies to gain control over thoughts and emotions. You may start feeling better by utilizing willingness, but willingness is not about trying to feel better. Willingness is about choosing to be in control of your life, instead of letting feelings control you. If you want to live fully, with all your experiences, pleasant and unpleasant, from your heart and your mind, you need to be willing. Willing to experience whatever there is to experience in your life. So that you can take steps in the direction you truly want to go, with your head and heart aligned.

Take a moment to check in with yourself and see how it feels to be invited to embrace full willingness.

Case Sophie: part 2

Early in therapy, I asked Sophie to write down her rules for herself and her children. Rules that she has for everyone to follow. Sophie found this exercise pleasant, and it made her feel good. She believes that life is good and, more importantly, that she is a good mother if everyone follows these rules. When I asked if she ever manages to adhere to all the rules, she said she does her best. However, it often doesn't work out, especially with her oldest child who frequently breaks the rules. I asked Sophie if she is willing to strictly follow all the rules she sets for herself and explored how that feels for her. In the following session, Sophie returned feeling sad. She had not been able to adhere to all her own rules, and it felt terrible for her.

Gradually, Sophie began to realize that she sets impossible demands for herself and for others, including her children. This realization triggered many emotions. We took several sessions to acknowledge and address these feelings. Sophie experienced anger toward herself for imposing such impossible demands on her children and sadness over the pressure she had put on herself for years. We oscillated between experiencing these emotions and discussing the workability and unworkability of rules. I frequently made remarks like, "Yes, this is challenging," "Yes, this is what you do," and "Yes, this is sad." These comments provided recognition and helped Sophie experience her emotions.

Sophie became increasingly willing to examine her own behavior and its impact on her children. She was willing to be more flexible with the rules to see what happens. She quickly noticed that her oldest child responded better to this approach. Sophie found therapy to be quite confronting because it allowed her to look at herself differently. She mentioned that she still loses her temper with her oldest child sometimes. Although she still does not like this, it has become more acceptable for her. Sophie has learned to view herself as a whole, enabling her to take responsibility for her behavior.

Summary and conclusion

In this chapter, we explored the concept of acceptance, which we prefer to refer to as "willingness." Willingness involves seeing and acknowledging what is present in your life at this very moment. To do so, you must be willing to look at it. We used metaphors such as yin and yang and the left and right sides of our bodies to illustrate the importance of looking at ourselves and our experiences as a whole. This includes both pleasant and unpleasant aspects of ourselves and our lives. Willingness also involves actively embracing experiences that we may prefer to keep at bay.

We emphasized the importance of therapists gaining their own experience with willingness in their personal lives. This allows them to empathize better with their clients and understand the challenges involved in this work. It also helps therapists recognize their own humanity, acknowledging that they have good and bad days and possess both admirable and flawed qualities. It is about being willing to be where you are, both as a human being and as a therapist, and accepting that you have knowledge and still have much to learn.

In our work with clients, it is essential that we are willing to meet them where they are. There is often pressure from society and even from within ourselves to push clients to be somewhere other than where they currently are in their journey. However, in therapy, the client determines the pace at which they are willing to confront their pain. The client is responsible for their life and the consequences of their behavior. As therapists, it can be challenging to accept and respect their chosen pace.

We demonstrated how acceptance and willingness can be applied using metaphors and exercises. It became evident that the various components of ACT are interconnected and cannot be isolated from each other. The key to working with acceptance and willingness is to also be competent in working with present moment, self-as-context and defusion.

Both therapists and clients experience fluctuations in their willingness. This is perfectly normal and should be recognized when either party's willingness is low. Willingness is about coming as close as possible to your pain, as far as it is feasible at the moment. Avoiding pain is a natural and understandable reaction. However, being willing to see everything that is present, whether pleasant or not, allows you to look at yourself as a whole and make choices accordingly. This enables you to move in the direction you desire.

Reference

Hayes, S. C., Strosahl, K. D., & Wilson, K. G. (1999). *Acceptance and commitment therapy: An experiential approach to behavior change*. New York: The Guilford Press.

Chapter 7

Letting go of your story and taking control of your life from self-as-context

Roy Thewissen

This chapter is about how you, as a therapist, together with your client can gradually cross the bridge from self-as-content to self-as-context. Most acceptance and commitment therapy (ACT) therapists find it difficult to work with self-as-context. Two questions arise during supervision. Firstly, what exactly is meant by this theoretically difficult concept? And secondly, how can you, as the therapist, effectively use self-as-context interventions within an ACT treatment? We will show in a comprehensible way that you can understand the concept of self-as-context as 'the behavior of perspective taking.' We explain what we mean by this and how your client can learn this behavior. Subsequently, we discuss various ways of teaching your client to look at his experiences, his story about these experiences, and the history of these stories, from varying perspectives. In this way, he connects with his self-as-context. From this place, he can make conscious and flexible behavioral choices, letting go of his story and take his life in his own hands.

Case Anne: part 1

Anne is a 38-year-old woman with chronic pain complaints. She also suffers from mood swings, tension, and anxiety complaints (agitation, restlessness). She worries a lot and suffers from fear of failure. She works as a nurse and is currently on sick leave.

In previous phases of therapy, she gained insight into the content of her story as well as her related behavioral repertoire. Both at home and at work, she was constantly working hard, caring for others, and ignoring her own feelings and needs. She looked primarily to the needs and wishes of others. This behavior matched her story, in which 'being strong' emerged as the most important theme. She labeled contacting and expressing more vulnerable emotions as 'being weak'. Developing pain complaints made it impossible for her to be constantly strong and brought her into contact with a 'vulnerable and weak' side of herself.

Anne had learned from adverse experiences in her past (being bullied at school; living with an alcoholic and aggressive father; a protective mother; little recognition for her feelings and needs; coerced study choice) to make herself 'invisible'. She allowed herself 'to be' only if she was strong and made herself available to others.

DOI: 10.4324/9781032699691-8

Why it is important to understand self-as-context as perspective-taking

At the start of an ACT treatment, we confronted the client with the unworkability of acting on his story in his current living circumstances. Moreover, he learned to pay more attention to his painful feelings and increase his ability to distance himself from unhelpful or even sabotaging thoughts. He has also learned to anchor himself in the present moment. While he has taken the necessary steps to break free from his story and its influence on his behavior, this has not been sufficient to achieve sustainable behavioral change in the service of a meaningful and valuable life. Learning to take perspective on yourself is the next step. In this context, self-as-context work is fundamental.

Connecting with self-as-context is necessary to break free from ones story

With the introduction of self-as-context, we are taking a necessary next step. We want the client to realize that he can break free from the content of his story and that there is a broader, all-encompassing context in which this story takes place. This is not easy, as we are asking the client to question the utility of their entire story. Engaging in this confrontation is a daring undertaking. We touch on the core of someone's identity. This often meets with resistance from clients, who do not want or cannot simply give up their familiar story.

If I am not my story, my feelings, and/or my thoughts, 'who am I?' The client wonders. You take this question very seriously as a therapist, and you explore it further when you work with self-as-context. "Who are you really, if you are not your story with all your thoughts, feelings and (physical) sensations?" Answering this question is a process that we build up slowly and step by step.

Experiencing self-as-context through the behavior of perspective-taking

Being in touch with your self-as-context is described as a psychological experience in which you are detached from your thoughts, feelings, and physical sensations. You 'see' yourself as the conscious space within which these experiences take place. People who regularly practice observing, and detaching, from their own experiences – through mindfulness or other forms of meditation – may recognize this broader experience of consciousness. However, working with self-as-context does not aim to achieve or pursue this state of consciousness. It is important that people anchor themselves in the present moment and can relate to the content of all their experiences (and their story) in a conscious way. After all, ACT is not necessarily about what we experience, but mainly about what behavior we can change.

The underlying behavior analytical theory (Relational Frame Theory [RFT]) makes it clear that self-as-context is not only an experience but also a behavior. Without going into the technical details of RFT, we learn that we can essentially think of self-as-context as a perspective-taking behavior on yourself and your story (e.g. McHugh and Stewart, 2012). By perspective, we mean a place from which we can look at something else. Just as we can look from our eyes at an object (e.g., the book you are reading now) in the outside world, we will now also look at objects in the inner world (the story of your own thoughts, feelings, and physical sensations).

Connecting with the experience of his self-as-context, the client initially takes an observer perspective from which he can observe his inner world (the continuous flow of thoughts, feelings, and sensations) and from which he can also perceive through his senses in the outside world (the physical environment, situations, and events). The experience of self-as-context cannot therefore be separated from the behavior of perspective-taking.

So, taking the perspective of self-as-context is an action. It is about the behavior of taking perspective, from which your client can relate to himself and the content of his story in a different way. We show in this chapter how to gradually guide your client through learning and applying the complex behavior of perspective-taking. These steps are crucial for experiencing self-as-context and achieving sustainable behavioral change.

Your client learns to take a perspective

Your client knows how to anchor himself in the present moment (Chapter 6). Now we want him to experience that this is a special place from which he can gain perspective. To clarify this for your client, it may be helpful to provide the metaphor of writer and reader of your own book. We will return to this book metaphor regularly in this chapter to clarify the different methods of perspective-taking when connecting with the self-as-context.

The metaphor of being the writer and reader of your own book

Your whole life, all your experiences are described in a book (your story). It is your story. You live your life from and in that story. You completely agree with it. You wrote down every experience, every perception in your book, with the same writing style and same genre. However, during the treatment, you came to realize that your life was also dictated by this book. You distanced yourself from your book and began to realize that you were not only the writer but also the reader of your book. You no longer coincide with the content of your book. You realize that you can look at this book from a distance, and that there is a part of you that writes it, a part that watches it, and a part that reads it.

This metaphor helps to connect your client to a psychological place from which he can look at himself and his experiences. Your client learns that there is a perspective from which he can read the written content of his story. This is an important step so that the client can begin to experience themselves as separate from the content of their story.

In the coming paragraphs, we will show how you and your client can cross the bridge from self-as-content (story) to self-as-context (perspective). We do this by allowing your client to take perspective on their own experiences in different ways. In this way, the client connects with her self-as-context.

How can you cross the bridge from content to context?

Crossing the bridge from content to context is a major challenge for both clients and therapists. It requires a completely different way of relating to ourselves and our experiences than we are used to in our daily lives. Your client has already learned to separate himself from the content of his experiences (see Chapter 4). Now we are taking it a step further. On the one hand, we want to teach the client to relate to his experiences (the content of his story) in a different way, and on the other hand, to realize that he does this by taking perspective on his experiences. He crosses the bridge, from identifying with his experiences (story content), to the perspective (context) he takes upon his experiences.

In the following paragraphs, we will cross the bridge step by step. A first step in which we guide the client is to become aware of and get to know his experiences; a second step is seeing his experiences change from moment to moment; and in the third step, he can adopt his I-here-now perspective from which he can observe all his experiences.

Your client becomes aware and gets to know his experiences

Your client can make a distinction between the content of his book (his story) and himself as the reader of it. By this, we mean that he realizes that his story is written by the many experiences he has had in his life so far. He now realizes that he is not only the protagonist of his story but also the reader. Your client gets to know himself because he can consciously notice and name his experiences (content of his story). This is what is often called 'self-as-process' in ACT. The better your client can notice this ever-changing stream of experiences, the better he gets to know the influence of his story on his behavior and the more he distances himself from his experiences. Even more importantly, by repeatedly noticing and naming his experiences, he begins to distinguish between the content of his experiences and the perspective from which he looks at, notices, and names his experiences. The client begins to connect with this perspective.

From the start of the therapy, we have guided the client in learning to name his thoughts, feelings, and sensations. Thoughts are always referred to as thoughts, feelings as feelings, and sensations as sensations that the client 'has' and not which the client 'is'. This is a skill (behavior) that the client will increasingly adopt and master as the therapy progresses.

Let us see how you, as a therapist, can also develop more awareness of your own inner experiences. Early in my career as a therapist, I often let myself be guided by the automatic flow of thoughts and feelings. For example, I was affected by a client who showed resistance in therapy. I felt irritated and tried harder to convince her that I was right. This was obviously not conducive to the therapeutic relationship and the further course of the treatment. It is equally important for us as therapists that we are regularly aware of our own stream of thoughts and feelings during our sessions. This way we can be more aware of our (automatic) reactions and check whether they are helpful for our therapeutic contact and the direction we want to take with our client. In the following exercise, we invite you to notice the stream of your own thoughts and feelings.

Exercise

Consider a conversation or specific event with a client in which, afterwards, you felt that you had not responded in a helpful way. For example, irritation you felt when a client was constantly absorbed in her story and was telling it incessantly; or a client who sat facing away from you with her coat on and barely said anything.

Think about what your client evoked. What thoughts and feelings did you notice? Name these below:

I had the feeling of ....

....

....

....

I had the thought of ....

....

....

....

My response was (What did you do in interaction with this client?):

....

....

....

To respond more consciously in interaction with our client, we need to be aware of what the situation evokes in us and how we tend to respond. Then we can think about this consciously. So, we always try to pay attention to our own stream of thoughts and feelings (and our reactions to them). This way we can ultimately choose more consciously how we want to respond in interaction with our client.

Your client sees that his experiences change from moment to moment

When the client learns to notice and name his thoughts and feelings, he can become more aware that his inner experiences are constantly changing. So, he learns to be aware of his stream of thoughts and feelings from moment to moment. We see some overlap here with the skill of contacting with the present. While contacting with the present is more about helping the client to anchor in the present moment, the emphasis in self-as-process is on getting to know the stream of inner experiences and connecting with the perspective from which he can notice his inner experiences. He sees his experiences from the I-here-now perspective, as something that takes place from moment to moment and is always changing.

You can ask your client to regularly reflect on the variability of his experiences during conversations. We invite our clients to practice this frequently at home. This makes it a skill he can always fall back on. The following questions and subsequent metaphor ('the photo presentation') can help you to get your client to notice and name the variation and changeability of his experience during a conversation:

Example procedure: make yourself aware that you are not the same as the experience

The following questions can help the client see the variety and changeability of their experiences, and notice that there is an observer who stands back from the experience:

- What thoughts/feelings/sensations can you notice right now? And now…?
- Do you notice that they come, go, and come back?
- From where do you notice this?

Following these questions, you can have your client reflect on the following metaphor.

The photo-show metaphor

Someone who is on vacation takes a lot of photos of a walk at a beautiful place in nature. He walks around, taking one photo after another.

He consciously captures every moment with his camera. He notes that all the moments he captures are different. The moments come and go. At the same time, he also realizes that he is the one holding the camera and capturing all these moments.

Once home, the photographer wants to view all the recorded experiences of his trip. He sits on the couch and watches the photo show of his nature walk on TV. He notes that one photo after another appears and disappears, that other photos keep appearing on the screen and disappearing again. At that moment, he may notice that he is sitting on the couch and watching the photo show on the TV with some distance. It is then even easier to see that there is a photographer and photos, and that the two are not the same.

It can also be similar if you look at your own internal experiences.

A client who is stuck endlessly worrying about what 'stupid' things he said during his last meeting could use the questions in the example to see how his thoughts were running away with him. This caused him to distance himself from his thinking. He could notice and name the comings and goings of his thoughts. As a result, he was no longer so attached to its content.

As therapists, we can also regularly reflect on our own experiences and mention them during conversations with our clients. We model in our own behavior what we want our client to learn to do with their own experiences. For example, a therapist who is affected by listening to a client talk about abuse may notice that it makes her sad and angry. She can name these feelings and share them with the client. In doing so, she acknowledges the client's intense emotional experience. The therapist also shows that it is okay to be vulnerable and that, in this way, she can emotionally connect with another person with whom she shares her feelings.

The client can then begin to connect with the perspective from which he can notice the comings and goings of his experiences. This perspective is always anchored in the present moment, and we therefore call it the I-here-now perspective. We will now see how we can allow the client to make even more explicit connection with this I-here-now perspective.

Your client connects with his I-here-now perspective

The client often finds it difficult to experience his thoughts as something that is truly distant from himself. He is easily carried away by the content. For example, if a client strongly believes that he is stupid, in situations where he makes a mistake, he will quickly be carried away by the literalness of his conclusion: 'I am stupid'. A metaphor can help make this distinction even clearer.

The metaphor of the platform and the train carriages

A man wakes up on a moving train. He looks out the window and sees everything flashing by. He realizes that he is on a familiar train again. It is one he gets onto every time. This time he decides to get off at the next stop and let the train continue. He is now standing on the platform and watching the various carriages of the train pass by. This allows him to see very clearly that the train consists of carriages that all pass by one by one. It is a very long train that he mainly knows from the inside because he was always carried along by the train. Now he is standing on the platform outside the train, and he can see the different carriages very clearly. One after another comes and goes. The man is not on the train and is not carried away by it. He is standing on the platform, and he realizes that he can observe the train, with the comings and goings of the carriages.

   We can look at our own thoughts in the same way.

So, from the place or perspective of the platform, your client can notice his own thoughts, feelings, and physical sensations as a flow of experiences from moment to moment, without having to go along with their content. The platform represents his I-here-now perspective.

   Let us expand on this place (your I-here-now perspective) by highlighting it as the place from which you observe your experiences (thoughts, feelings, and sensations). By asking in different ways about 'who notices?' you can make an even clearer connection with your I-here-now perspective. The following exercise contains questions that can help both you as a therapist and your client to strengthen the connection with the I-here-now perspective. We ask you to reflect on these questions yourself to strengthen the I-here-now perspective and notice what they do in your own experience.

Exercise

We have already noted that you can see certain thoughts, which have always largely determined your behavior, as something separate from yourself. Now let us see how you can notice from where you are watching the comings and goings of your thoughts. Reflect on your experiences (thoughts and feelings) at this moment.

   Describe what you have experienced by considering the following questions:

- Can you notice that you are noticing?

- Can you notice that you are present all the time as your experience changes from moment to moment?
- Who holds the camera? Is the person holding the camera different from the photos you take?
- Do you realize that there is an 'I', here-and-now, who has these experiences and can observe, notice, and name them?

Briefly describe your experience:

....

....

....

....

....

....

....

If you explore your client's experiences in this way, it can give him the freedom to step out of his patterns. He can do this, for example, by ceasing the struggle against unwanted feelings and sensations or by not following the rules of his story. The added value is that he gets to know this psychological place, his I-here-now perspective, better and better. It is from this place that he can relate to the content of his story in a different way. The client will recognize this place himself and will continue connecting with this place. The client must be immersed in his experience and know this place inside and out.

As a therapist, it is important to slowly build up this process of awareness over many sessions (and throughout the entire treatment) and to keep coming back to it. We practice this way of taking perspective regularly during the sessions. For example, when the client talks about an emotionally charged experience and you notice that he (again) identifies with its content, you help him (again) to distance himself and, despite being emotionally affected, to connect with his I-here-now perspective. It is important to note here that the intention is not to necessarily make the client feel less. The function of self-as-context is to let the client experience that there is still a person and that this person has a feeling.

The following mini-transcript contains questions you can ask to help your client solidify his connection with his I-here-now perspective. It provides an example of how to help your client recognize the I-here-now perspective as the psychological place from which to view, notice, and name their emotional responses and experiences (thoughts, feelings, and sensations).

We invite you to read the transcript first and then do this exercise for yourself. To do this, consider a difficult situation (personal or professional). Put yourself in the client's place.

Mini transcript on connecting with an I-here-now perspective

Client:	It's been a rough week. I have completely lashed out at my children again. And even though they had hardly done anything. I feel really bad about it.
Therapist:	That's not nice to hear. I see it really touched you.
Client:	Yes, it really hit home. I really feel like I'm failing as a mother again.
Therapist:	That's a familiar conclusion, isn't it? Can you see that it touched you in that part of your story?
Client:	[remains silent for a moment]
Therapist:	Now let's look at from where you can start looking at this part of your story. From this place, you can look at the thoughts, feelings, and sensations that arise. It may help to close your eyes for a moment while you bring the situation back to mind.
Client:	Okay. [Client closes eyes]
	The therapist emphasizes connecting with the place (I-here-now perspective) from which the client can look at, notice, and name her experiences.
Therapist:	You are now back in the situation. Allow the reactions – thoughts, feelings, and sensations – to arise and notice them. You don't have to answer the questions I'm going to ask you. Just notice what they evoke in your experience.

As a therapist, you can ask, for example, the following questions:

• Can you notice that as you are thinking and speaking these thoughts, there is someone sitting there in that chair who can notice these thoughts?
• Can you hear your thoughts in your head? And then hear it while pronouncing it? Who is it that hears these thoughts?
• Realize that it is 'you', here-and-now, who can hear and notice these thoughts, feelings, and sensations. That you can watch these reactions in this situation from a distance.

Exercise

You can also ask the client to write down their thoughts, feelings, and sensations on post-its and place them in front of them. The therapist now emphasizes the place from which she looks at these experiences.

- Let's identify and write down what is going on in your head and body at this moment [write on different post-its].
  - Can you now look at these post-its from a distance?
  - Who is looking at these post-its?
  - Are you these post-its or are you the one looking at them?

Describe your own experience with the above questions:

....

....

....

....

....

....

....

....

....

....

During your sessions, you can regularly have your client look at his experiences in this way and thus promote connecting with his I-here-now perspective. We also ask the client to regularly contact his I-here-now perspective in a similar way in his home situation. In this way, the behavior of taking one's I-here-now perspective and learning to recognize this place can be acquired in a sustainable way.

Your client has learned to make a clear distinction between the content of his story (thoughts, feelings, and physical sensations) and his I-here-now perspective (context), from which he can consciously observe and name his experiences (content), and can see this as something that changes from moment to moment (self-as-process). This undermines the attachment to the content of his story. Your client will feel freer from the impact of his story on his behavior.

Your client has now crossed the bridge from coinciding with the content of his story and all his experiences to connecting with the context in which these experiences take place and from which he can observe and name them (I-here-now perspective). This perspective is what we call self-as-context in ACT. The concepts of self-as-context and the I-here-now perspective used in this chapter are synonyms of each other. Next, we see how the client can further deepen and strengthen his connection with his self-as-context (I-here-now perspective).

Your client becomes the 'owner' of his self-as-context

Your client has learned to connect with his I-here-now perspective. He can recognize when he is led by the content of his story or when he connects with a place from which he can observe the content of his story. However, it is not enough for your client to recognize when he is in his observer perspective. We want him to be able to make conscious and more free choices to regain governance over his life. This requires that your client can easily connect with his self-as-context or take this position when he notices that he is being lived by his story again. Metaphorically speaking, we can say that your client should become the owner of this place. This is like owning your own home with all the furniture and personal belongings in it.

How can your client further strengthen his connection with his self-as-context? We will allow your client to take ownership of his self-as-context by experiencing this place as (1) an overarching and all-encompassing container for the content of his story and (2) as a perspective from which to look at his own story throughout his lifecycle.

Experiencing self-as-context as an overarching all-encompassing container

Through frequent practice of the previous steps, your client has become familiar with the stability of his self-as-context. He can observe the content of his own story without being constantly determined by it. Space has been created between himself as a perspective, i.e., the reader of his story, and the written content of his story.

We will now take a further step in fostering his self-as-context. It is very easy for people to coincide with their story again and, therefore, let it determine their behavior. It is often a pitfall for ACT counselors to want to continue with the treatment at this point too quickly. However, your client's contact with his self-as-context is crucial to learning to deal with the inevitable relapse into the behavioral patterns of his story. ACT is about learning to choose behavior that is helpful for a values-oriented life in a conscious and flexible way. This requires your client to become very familiar with his I-here-now perspective. And that in turn requires the therapist to pay systematic and ample attention to promoting self-as-context in the client.

The growing awareness of 'I am not my story' brings the client into contact with some special qualities of this perspective. From this place, he can experience that he is more and bigger than his story (including the content of thoughts, feelings, sensations, conclusions, beliefs, etc.) and that he encompasses all parts of this content, like a large container. A container is more than and larger than its contents. A container includes and contains everything that is in it. All parts of the content are carried by the container, regardless of what those parts are.

These qualities of self-as-context are crucial for the client to truly stay out of the content of his story. For example, an anxious client who is confronted with criticism of her work learns that she can simultaneously experience feelings and thoughts of her fear of rejection and observe and name them from a distance. She 'carries' all these anxious thoughts and feelings in her 'overarching and all-encompassing container'. She is the container of all her experiences: the positive, the negative; the desired as well as the undesirable. As a container, she is more than and greater than the content of all her (fearful) experiences. As a container, she encompasses and contains all her (anxious) experiences. From "the contact-with-the-container quality" of her self-as-context, there is room to stay out of the usual behavioral patterns of her story and ultimately to respond differently in this situation.

One way to help your client experience the overarching and all-encompassing qualities of their self-as-context is to regularly use metaphorical language in conversations. This can help your client to place his experiences within his self-as-context as a container of all his experiences (the content of his story). We would like to ask you to think about this yourself and consider the following analogies when looking at your own experiences.

Self-as-context analogies

- Do you notice that all your experiences are part of a bigger picture?
- You are like a container that contains and encompasses everything within it.
- After all, you are more than and greater than all your experiences from your present, past, and future.
- All your experiences are part of your conscious I-here-now.

Your client experiences that he can relate to the content of his experiences (story) in a fundamentally different way. He now experiences that he is even the 'owner' of all his experiences that he carries with him in his broader container perspective. His story, with all its content, is part of him as an overarching and all-encompassing container.

We want the client to be able to use his self-as-context in his daily life. After all, it is the current context in which he is confronted with his story that determines how he responds to all kinds of difficult situations. Introducing a metaphor can help the client to connect with his self-as-context. The following metaphor expands on the 'writer and reader of your book' metaphor (see beginning of this chapter) and emphasizes the quality of an "overarching and all-encompassing container" perspective.

The metaphor of the librarian of all your books

(This metaphor builds on the previous writer and reader metaphor)

You have had many experiences during your life and described them in many books. You have come to realize that you are the writer and reader of your books (your story) and that you can therefore look at your books from a distance. This perspective already made you less identified with the content of your story. Now we can go one step further.

You could say that every person has a whole library full of books (or stories from their history). In all those books, the leading role is played by the person whose life it is about. Looked at this way, you could say that a person is not only the writer and reader of all his books, but that he indeed is the librarian of the entire library. A librarian is the owner of all the books in the library.

Imagine if that also applied to all the books you have lived and written throughout your life. Let us explore how you can further develop this librarian perspective on yourself and your story, and whether it can help you relate differently to what you are facing in your life. What would it mean if you became the librarian?

From this metaphor, your client can experience that he is the broader perspective within which his story takes place. As a writer and reader of his own life story, he sees that there are more books – not just his current story, but even a whole bookcase, a whole library full of books and stories. He had previously made the transition from being stuck in the story of a book as a writer to being a reader of his book (self-as-process). Now he is making the transition to being the owner (librarian) of all the books in his library. This is the broadest and most free way to take perspective on himself and his story.

In the next section, we will see how we can help the client relate to the history of his story in a different way. This can further strengthen ownership of his story and create space to choose more consciously and freely how he wants to act (see later in this chapter).

Let your client look at himself during his lifecycle

It is not enough for your client to 'free himself' from the content of his story and encompass it in a broader overarching perspective. His story has a past that largely dictates his present, and if he remains blind to this, it will also determine his future.

As discussed earlier, the many books in his library describe his life and, in addition to the many conclusions and beliefs, all kinds of 'rules' about how he should or should not behave. Take, for example, a client who has derived a general rule from the conclusion "I am worthless": "I should always be nice to other people."

This rule can elicit behavior in relevant situations, such as always saying yes to requests, gauging the expectations of others, and attempting to meet them. Without perhaps realizing it, the client repeats the behavioral strategies learned from his past. In other words, how your client responds to current situations is (largely) determined by how he has learned to respond in the past (see Chapter 2). He is thus trapped in his story, which keeps repeating itself in changing life circumstances but with similar behavioral strategies.

To be able to choose more freely here-and-now, he must free himself from the influence of the story of his past on his current behavior. Of course, he can no longer change his past, but he can change his relationship to the story about that past. The client has now learned to see himself as the context of his story (self-as-context; the librarian). From this perspective, he can look at his past in a different way and change his relationship to it. This gives him more space to make choices other than those dictated by his past (his story).

As a therapist, we can help the client to take a different perspective on his life history. We want to empower the client in his self-as-context by emphasizing that this is broader than the stories that younger versions of himself have collected throughout his life and that his self-as-context includes all of these (and more). One option to do this with your client is to use a 'physical' metaphor: 'seeing yourself during your life'. By a physical metaphor, we mean that you are going to do something with your client in the physical space. In this case, you have your client stand in different positions to physically express what you are instructing with words. This metaphor can help him to better understand who he was at the time and what he experienced at the time.

We would like to ask you to experience this metaphor yourself. First, read the following exercise completely, and then take the time to perform it. Afterwards, write down what you experienced while doing this exercise.

Exercise: seeing yourself during your life (physical metaphor)

Write the following ages on three sheets of paper: 10 years, 20 years, and your current age. Arrange these sheets in a timeline from left to right, starting with the youngest age. If necessary, find a few photos of these ages and add them.

Then take plenty of time to recall a memory appropriate for the different ages. Choose a relatively neutral or positive memory.

Stand upright and take the different positions by standing on the sheets of paper (with age). With every position you take, you put yourself back in the memory of your younger version ('you-then-there'). You look from here-and-now at what you experienced then and there.

Start with the sheet of your current age. Stand on the sheet with the ages of 10 and 20 years and end up back on the sheet of your current age. Just look at what comes to mind without doing anything else with it. Just notice and observe. As you take on the different positions, you can consider some reflective questions:

- What is it like to see through the eyes of yourself at this age/this moment?
- What thoughts, feelings, and sensations arise?
- Reflect on your experience that you are aware here-and-now of what you were aware of at that moment (10/20 years) and are aware of now (present moment).

Realize that you are seeing and experiencing through the eyes of your 10-year-old/20-year-old/present self. 'I am here-and-now; I think …; I feel …; I feel in my body…'

When you return to your present age, open your eyes and step back (or stand on a chair) so that you can see the entire timeline (10 years, 20 years, present age). Reflect on some qualities of your overarching and all-encompassing container perspective (self-as-context).

- I-here-now I always have been, and I always will be. In my past, my present, and my future, whatever I have experienced, I am experiencing now and will continue to experience. Always from the perspective of I-here-now.
- I am more than/greater than/contain and encompass all my experiences in my past, present, and future.
- All my experiences, in my past, present, and future, are part of me; I-here-now.

I can choose what behavior I exhibit and what direction I want to take with my life now and in the future.

Now that you have performed this exercise, we ask you to write down what you experienced during this exercise.

Write down your experiences

What was it like to take on the position of your younger self again (as a 10- and 20-year-olds)?

....

....

....

....

....

What was it like to experience all of your experiences (past and present) from an I-here-now perspective?

....

....

....

....

....

What was it like to experience yourself as an 'overarching all-encompassing container'?

....

....

....

....

....

When you apply this metaphor as a therapist, it is important not to respond to the content of the story that the client comes up with. The content itself is not important in this phase. The client knows his story to a certain extent, can look at it from a distance and see that he is not the same as it. After the exercise, you ask about the experiences he has had while taking different perspectives. Below, we give an example of what such a debriefing could look like.

Mini transcript about the debriefing of the previous exercise

Therapist: What was it like for you to look at your experiences from different positions?

Client:	That was nice. When I was ten years old, I still felt like a free child and had few worries.
Therapist:	That's nice. I'm especially curious about what it was like to go back to your younger version of ten years from your I-here-now perspective. What was that like for you?
Client:	I thought it was special that I could see my ten-year-old self. How she was then and how I felt then.
Therapist:	So, you were able to move to the place of 'you' as a ten-year-old and be aware of what you were aware of at the time?
Client:	Yes, indeed, it was like traveling back in time and seeing my younger self again.
Therapist:	What was it like to look back at your younger versions from the perspective I-here-now and see that you have always looked through your eyes from I-here-now?
Client:	Yes, I have always experienced everything in the present moment, as things kept happening and I grew older. I have always been me... that somehow feels like something stable and gives confidence or something... I don't know how to explain it. It feels good to be in this conscious place.
Therapist:	What was it like to step back and see your entire lifecycle at a glance and experience that you are more and bigger than all your versions so far?
Client:	In a way that felt very liberating. As if I was completely disconnected from myself and could see myself from a distance throughout my life. Like looking down from a mountain and seeing the entire valley. It made me feel calm. And yes, as if I am more than all those younger 'Me's' in my life.

We especially take the time to reflect on the experiences of the last step, where the client experiences the self-as-context position. What you want to convey to your client is that he can see that he always has experienced all his experiences during his life, from an I-here-now perspective. This metaphor can promote the experience of the stability of self-as-context. We want our client to realize that there is always an overarching, all-encompassing I-here-now perspective (self-as-context) that he can connect with, even during the stormy moments in his life when he is swept away by the content of the story.

You can regularly return to the experiences during this exercise during the following sessions of the treatment. We also invite the client to reflect at home on what it is like to realize that his behavior (or strategies) has emerged from his story and its history and, above all, to regularly connect with his self-as-context as an overarching, all-encompassing container.

In the next part, we see that the client is 'freer' to choose from his connection with his self-as-context as an overarching, all-encompassing container. In the next chapter, we will explore with the client which of his behavioral patterns he does or does not want to continue in order to continue his life in a valuable way.

Learning to choose consciously from self-as-context

Now that your client can make full contact with his self-as-context, he is in a (psychological) place where he can look with a broad perspective at how the story of his life has partly determined how he is now stuck in his life. He can take perspective on the content of his story – with a past, present, and potential future. In this place, he is more distanced from his 'old' story, and his past no longer completely determines his present and future.

From this perspective, new behavioral choices are possible. The client can now consciously choose behavior that contributes to a meaningful life for him. The client's new behavioral choices will often contradict the conclusions and beliefs from his 'old' story. For example, he chooses to take the initiative in establishing new friendships. This may go against his belief that he is not worth it, and that people think he is stupid and boring.

It is now possible for all his old and gradually formed new conclusions and beliefs to coexist and integrate them into the overarching container perspective of his self-as-context. He is the owner of all his thoughts, feelings, sensations, conclusions, and beliefs; of his 'old' story with all its rules that he has always lived by, as well as the new, more flexible rules about how he wants to behave now and in the future. We want to help the client to choose new behavior more freely from his self-as-context.

Your client wonders who he actually wants to be

As your client becomes more detached from his story, he realizes that the story he has lived for a long time no longer works in his current living conditions. Sometimes your client even realizes that the story he has been living is not the story that was really his story. He realizes that he was lived by others and by circumstances. Maybe he will conclude that he was mostly just surviving. It is not surprising that in this phase of the therapy there is a shift from the question 'Who was I?' to the question 'Who do I actually want to be?'

First of all, we want our client to feel that he has a choice about his behavior. That he should no longer be the puppet of his story, even though that story will always remain part of his library.

Can your client choose something other than his old story?

Your client is the librarian of his library with all its books. He experiences himself as the owner of his story, and he can encompass its content in an overarching way (container perspective). In working with ACT, as with many other forms of therapy, it is not sufficient for your client to gain insights about himself and his lifecycle. He comes to therapy because he is stuck in his life and wants something different. Breaking free from the struggle with himself frees your client to tackle the challenges in his life differently here-and-now. So, it requires different or new behavior.

The broad perspective of self-as-context offers your client the chance to find inspiration and motivation for new behavior. Your client can now learn to choose differently than the patterns (content) of his old story dictate. For example, your client realizes that his behavior has been guided by his old story ('I am unimportant and it is better to be invisible in contact with others') to constantly put himself in the background (e.g., not saying much about himself in a group, choosing work where he has little contact with other people or to behave docilely within a team, or always letting others go first in a queue at the cash register).

On the other hand, it provides a context for your client to consciously make more free and more flexible choices. Regardless of what those choices are, we teach our client to consciously choose certain behaviors and its consequences (as far as they can be foreseen). He can therefore consciously choose to exhibit behavior that deviates from the core beliefs of his old story (for example, to speak out more about his feelings and needs in a group, to take more initiative in his work, to choose whether or not to give someone priority at the cash register). He might also choose, faced with feelings of fear, to avoid expressing himself. Whatever he chooses, he does so from his self-as-context, with his eyes open, realizing the consequences of his behavior. ACT treatment is about helping your client exercise governance of his life (again) and learn to choose behavior that helps him to live his life in a meaningful way.

This conscious choice for something different (or the same) than the old story touches the foundations of his identity. The client may wonder: Was and am I the person I want to be? In the previous example, the client may wonder whether he still wants to continue as someone who goes through life 'invisibly'. Or does he now want to take steps in which he will make himself increasingly 'visible' and choose a behavioral repertoire that is an expression of this? The question of 'who I was/am' makes room for the question 'who do I want to be/become'. From his self-as-context, his identity (his story about who he is and what he does) is not determined solely by external circumstances but can now also be driven by conscious, self-considered choices. We try to strengthen our client's capacity to exercise governance over his behavioral choices, regardless of the dominance of his old story. One possibility is to provide the following metaphor.

The metaphor of the horse-drawn carriage

Imagine a carriage pulled by two horses. Both horses can pull the carriage in a different direction. And the coachman may then be at the mercy of the dominance of one horse in one direction or the other horse choosing another direction. However, he can also take the reins from the carriage and determine for himself in which direction the carriage moves. But even if the coachman takes the reins himself, the direction is not completely free to choose. The landscape helps determine which roads are more or less passable and which obstacles the coachman must overcome. The horses can also still run wild and pull the carriage in a different direction than the coachman wants.

It is the same with our stories. They do not disappear, and they can always pull us along. The extent to which this is possible depends on the extent to which we exercise governance of the reins ourselves. That often takes time and practice.

A similar metaphor in ACT is 'the bus metaphor' (Hayes et al., 1999), which was already described in the chapter on defusion. Here, the client, as the driver, is the one who holds the steering wheel and can always decide by which passengers he will or will not be guided, when steering his bus in a direction he wants to go. He takes the passengers in his bus in the direction he chooses, instead of being taken by the whims of the passengers (the conclusions and beliefs of his old story). He always chooses from his I-here-now perspective (self-as-context). Behavioral choices are therefore anchored in the here-and-now. Only in the present moment can he show different behavior with his arms, legs, and vocal cords. Thoughts and feelings are like fellow travelers on his bus who can only have their say. It is up to him (as driver) to listen to their say or not. He sits at the wheel and controls the direction he takes the bus (his life).

Case Anna: part 2

In the framework of self-as-context, I first practiced with Anna distinguishing between the content of her story and her as a writer and reader of her story. After introducing this metaphor, we examined her various difficult situations during several sessions. She learned to notice and name her own (inner) reactions to these situations. For example, she might notice that when her daughter asked to watch over the children, she felt tension in her stomach and throat and a fear of hurting her daughter if she did not agree. She noticed that the anxiety quickly decreased, but that she also ignored her own need for rest. Over the course of several sessions, she could see her thoughts, feelings, and sensations coming and going; and that she could notice and name these from a distance (self-as-process).

By viewing this with her as a photo show, photo by photo, and letting her approach her experiences from the perspective of the person in the chair looking at the photos, she made the link with herself as a reader of her own story. She connected with her I-here-now perspective (as an observer). She further became familiar with this (psychological) place by practicing at home with the metaphor of 'the platform and the train carriages' and applying it to all kinds of experiences, for example, when she went for a walk or watched her children play.

She found stability in her I-here-now perspective by continually returning to her observational perspective during the sessions, when she talked about emotionally intense experiences with her partner and children.

We strengthened her connection with her self-as-context by practicing with the overarching container perspective during the session. This perspective was repeatedly touched upon by allowing her to experience, using (metaphorical) language, that she is more and greater than the content of all her experiences. From this perspective, she also began to look at some major life events in her past that contributed to creating the conclusions, beliefs, and behavior patterns of her story, where she now finds herself stuck. She put her life story into perspective and could see from a distance how, through her experiences in her family of origin, she started to focus on the needs and wishes of others. How attention to her own feelings and needs were ignored and misunderstood. She realized that she had learned behavior focused on caring for others and working hard all the time, both at home and at work, and how this shaped her story of 'being strong'. She recognized how fear of being weak, failing, or not doing well in the eyes of others led her to put herself at the service of others, at the expense of her own feelings and needs. She connected more with the pain of missing out on the loving care and attention for herself.

Anna could experience that there was a continuity of her I-here-now perspective in both the difficult and beautiful moments of her life history. It inspired her to give her life a new turn and no longer to be guided by her 'being strong' story. The metaphor of 'the librarian of all your books' helped her to take ownership of her own story and to recognize which behaviors of hers were determined by this. Furthermore, it helped her to reconnect with her self-as-context during difficult situations within her family.

She began to see that she had a choice in the present moment, as she no longer identified with her stories (books) in her library. The feeling of being able to choose was promoted by the metaphor of 'the driver and the horse cart'. Anna was given the reins back in her hands and was able to choose more consciously which horse/story she was guided by (being allowed to be strong or also allowed to be vulnerable). For example, when in contact with her daughter, she sincerely showed her vulnerability and was able to clearly indicate that she could no longer look after her children for as long or as often in order to have more time to take care of herself.

Summary and conclusions

During her ACT treatment, the client started to experience more 'distance' from her (painful) thoughts, feelings, and sensations. She also came to realize that certain conclusions, beliefs, and rules strongly determined her behavior and that she had been stuck within her story. She realized that she has lived most of her life through this story. She went to therapy because she wanted 'something different' with her life. For this purpose, it was not enough to free herself from just isolated (unwanted) parts of her story, but it was also necessary to break free from its entire content. This required a radical shift in how she viewed herself. The question 'Who was and am I?' gradually shifted to 'Who do I want to be?' for her life now and in the future.

In this chapter, we have seen how clients can learn to adopt a new perspective where they can relate in a fundamentally different way to the story that, up until now, has largely determined their behavior. They have learned to distance themselves from the content of that story and have crossed over to an overarching, all-encompassing self-as-context, as a broader perspective from which more conscious and free choices are possible.

During the gradual crossing, we begin by allowing clients to experience, on the one hand, noticing (or observing) and naming their flow of thoughts, feelings, and sensations, and on the other hand, seeing their changeability (self-as-process). More importantly, we emphasize getting them in touch with their I-here-now perspective from which they can do this. The metaphorical method of questioning, as well as metaphors such as 'writer and reader of your book' and 'the platform and the train carriages', help clients to connect with the self-as-context (I-here-now perspective).

It is not enough for your client to recognize when he is in contact with his self-as-context and, from there, to observe his own inner reactions. He must fully own this psychological place and take ownership of the content of his story. Once again, as a therapist, you can use (metaphorical) language to let your client experience that she is more than and bigger than her story (including the content of thoughts, feelings, sensations, conclusions, beliefs, etc.). Another important quality of self-as-context that the client comes to know is that it contains or encompasses all parts of this content in one large container. These qualities highlight the overarching and all-encompassing nature of his self-as-context and are expressed in the metaphor of the "librarian of all your books." By using a physical metaphor ('seeing yourself during your life'), your client can see how his past largely determines his actions in the present. At the same time, this metaphor promotes his self-as-context as an I-here-now perspective from which he can include and encompass the history and progression of his life story. He is now firmly anchored in his self-as-context.

As the owner of his own life story, the client can exercise governance of his life again. His past no longer must dictate his present and potential future. He is in a psychological place from which he can more consciously and freely choose to adjust his behavior or give it a different direction. He also finds inspiration in this place to reflect on important questions: What do you want your life to be about? What is really important and valuable in your life? Who do you want to be in relation to yourself and significant others? These and other questions will motivate your client to consciously choose behavior, from his self-as-context, in the service of a life that is valuable to him. In the next chapter, we will discuss these questions.

References

Hayes, S. C., Strosahl, K. D., & Wilson, K. G. (1999). Acceptance and commitment therapy: An experiential approach to behavior change. Guilford Press.

McHugh, L., & Stewart, I. (2012). The self and perspective taking: Contributions and applications from modern behavioral science. Oakland: New Harbinger Publications.

Chapter 8

Values-oriented action from self-as-context

Roy Thewissen

In this chapter, we offer you tools to explore together with your client what gives his life meaning and value, for now and in the future. As a result of being anchored in his 'I-here-now' perspective (self-as-context; Chapter 7), the client is connected to a psychological place from which he can make more conscious and free choices. He no longer must follow the whims of his story (self-as-content, Chapter 2) and can regain governance over his life path. In order to find life direction, it is important that your client discovers what is valuable to him and in which direction he wants to move. We will see how you can help your client with the challenge of behaving in line with his values again and again, even if he is seduced by his story again. The question from the previous chapter. 'Who am I?' shifts in this chapter to 'Who do I actually want to be?'

Case Lisa: part 1

Lisa reports she experiences insecurity, lots of worrying, anxiety attacks, and a general feeling of sadness, and a lack of zest for life. She avoids contact with people she does not know well, especially in larger groups. When she does meet up with people, she feels uncomfortable and tends to stay in the background. She has a solo job as a laboratory technician, where she can mainly use her technical skills. She generally thinks that people find her weird and not interesting to be around.

She adopts an 'invisible' attitude toward others based on this belief. She has always placed herself in the background in her social life and only becomes visible in her intellectual life, previously at school and now at work. Furthermore, she has always experienced a feeling of unease, a sense of not really belonging anywhere, and loneliness. As a sport, she always goes cycling alone. She enjoys reading exciting thrillers and cooking when she is at home in the evenings.

What are values and how are they linked to committed action?

Exploring the question 'Who do I actually want to be?' arises from the work we have already done on self-as-context in Chapter 7. To answer this question, we

DOI: 10.4324/9781032699691-9

want the client to reflect on what would make his life valuable if, unhindered by his story and its history, he could choose to act in the service of his values.

First, we want to clarify what we mean by values and how they are linked to committed action. And secondly, how your client can let his behavior be guided by what really matters to him instead of depending on whether or not he achieves a goal or result.

How are values linked to committed action?

You may be reading this book because you think it is important to further explore and train yourself in acceptance and commitment therapy (ACT). Values are abstract concepts such as deepening learning, emotional connection, trust, honesty, or togetherness, which refer to something that is meaningful and valuable in our lives and gives direction to our actions. In other words, what does your client want his life to be about, and what makes this important or valuable to him. For example, a client no longer wants to be guided by his fear of rejection because he finds it valuable to engage in more emotionally profound contacts.

This shows that values and committed actions are closely linked. We will therefore further discuss values-oriented action. We say that a certain behavior is values-oriented if it contributes to living according to your values. We will do or continue to do a certain behavior more often if this behavior gives us something we want to have or achieve (goal- or result-oriented behavior). We humans can also perform behavior that contributes to something that is personally meaningful or valuable to us. In other words, values are about the motivation of behavior, about why you do something. It is important that value-oriented action arises from one's own choice and is not merely following rules imposed or instructed by others. In ACT, we prefer to be guided by our values rather than focusing on achieving a specific goal or outcome.

Preferring values-oriented action over goal- or result-oriented action

Both clients and therapists usually become enthusiastic when they get to work with values. The client can deduce that he can now change something and that he can achieve a certain goal or result with it. He usually also expects that this will lead to pleasant feelings. For example, with 'honesty' as an important value in the partner relationship, the client may want to share her vulnerable feelings more: 'I feel sad because I notice that you are not at home much and at work a lot.' What is valuable here is about much more than the result or consequence of this behavior. The client may hope that her partner will make more time to spend together and that he will not become angry if she speaks out. However, value-oriented action is about what makes this behavior valuable for the client himself, such as honesty in communication, daring to show vulnerability, and showing more of oneself.

These values can be a strong impetus (motivation) to express more her feelings and needs. The values of 'honesty, vulnerability, and visibility' are about *why* she does it. And just performing the behavior ('sharing vulnerable feelings') is valuable in itself. In other words, doing the behavior and *why* it is done is what is important and valuable. What her behaviors 'yield' is then secondary. Of course, it is nice if the partner responds with understanding and will make more time for her, but value-oriented action does not depend on this.

Values are therefore not (positive) feelings, and value-oriented action is not goal- or result-oriented. This makes values in working with ACT so special. Values are self-chosen life directions on matters that matter in our client's life, and these can at all times encourage values-oriented action. As therapists, we want to continually prioritize and stimulate this.

The fact that the client learns to choose things that matter in his life, without making this depend on a predetermined goal or result, is important for two reasons. First, it can motivate the client to perform the behavior regardless of the difficult thoughts and feelings that arise before, during, and after performing the behavior (acceptance). He can invest again and again in behavior that contributes to what he finds valuable in his life. So not focused on a result in the client's inner world. Secondly, we want the client to take back governance over the direction of their life path, regardless of the vagaries of existence or the elusive reactions of others. So it is not dependent on the result in the client's outside world.

How does your client want his life to continue?

This question naturally arises when the client has learned to look at himself, his life, and his behavior from the perspective of his self-as-context (the librarian metaphor). He can distance himself from the story of himself and is less guided by difficult and painful thoughts and feelings. He has insight into part of the history and development of certain patterns in his life. The main themes of his story have become clearer. He can see which conclusions, beliefs, and associated behavioral patterns prevent him from living the life he would like. The client reflects on what really matters in his life and explores which behavior is useful for a life, here and now, that is meaningful and valuable to him.

We start exploring his value-oriented actions from being anchored in self-as-context by returning to the metaphor of 'the librarian' and expanding it further. In this metaphor, the client is at a place from which he can start investigating how he wants his life to continue, who he actually wants to be, and which behavioral choices are worth investing in. We invite you to reflect on this metaphor and associated questions before presenting this exercise to clients.

The metaphor of your life as a librarian (extension)

You could see your life as a story of many experiences and events that you have described in many books. They are all in your library. You have come to realize that you are not only the writer and reader of all your books (your story), but that you can also be the librarian.

The librarian is the owner and holder of all the books in his library. As a librarian, he is separate from the written content of all these books. He can read any book and put it back again. The books do not determine what the librarian does in his life. He can make conscious and free choices in his life.

You have been living your story for many years and have now come to the point of putting your feet in a different direction. Every moment in your life is a new moment and offers the opportunity to take a different path and acquire new experiences.

What would it be like to live your life as a librarian?

What would it be like, from the position of librarian, to consider the following important questions:

Where do you want your life to go?

What do you want your life to be about?

What makes your life meaningful and valuable?

And above all, who do you want to be in your life, now and in the future?

By exploring these questions from the position of a librarian, you can discover which behavior you want to choose that contributes to what you find important and valuable in your life, regardless of whether that is as expected or disappointing. You have taken back governance of your life, and you create what you find meaningful and valuable. In this way, you take steps to become who you want to be.

Based on this metaphor, the client can derive and realize that as a librarian, he is in a place from which he is aware of his story and its impact on his life. He now has insight into his life as he has lived it so far and can identify which behaviors contributed to him getting stuck. Working with self-as-context creates space and curiosity for the client to focus on the present and the future. He can find inspiration in his life story – his past and present – to decide for himself how he wants his life to continue.

In the next paragraph, we see that the pain of missing or having lost something that is meaningful to the client is a direct entrance to what is valuable to him for his life now and in the future. We will then see how we can deepen the client's reflection on and contact with his values in an experience-oriented manner. This is necessary so that the client can commit to a new and flexible behavioral repertoire.

Finding values in the pain of missing or losing something valuable

Only later in life did I find the love of my life and become a father. All those years before, I doubted whether I was worthy to share a life with someone, let alone start a family. I saw all my friends find partners, have children, and raise them together. I then experienced very strongly how important my values are – such as deep emotional connection, being able to care for someone else, being really seen and really seeing someone else, sharing life together – are for me. During my own professional development, I learned to take a broader perspective on my life development, and I came into contact with the pain of this loss. I could see how conclusions and beliefs from my past (my story) caused me to avoid contact with this pain and related values. I was stuck, and life was passing me by. My life history is indelible, and I carry it with me. It was only when I dared to connect with the pain of missing this precious thing that I could learn to do something other than stay stuck in avoidance and follow the conclusions of my story.

Our clients can also become aware of certain things that they have missed in their life development. For example, the lack of learning to stand up for themselves or having barely learned to take their feelings and needs into account. It may also be that the client has lost things valuable to him. For example, after the death of a partner, losing a job, or being confronted with physical limitations. These and many similar experiences provide the client and therapist with fertile ground to explore their values.

In the following dialogue, we show how the therapist brings the client into contact with what she has missed in her past. And how this can serve as inspiration to gain further insight into which values can serve as a guideline for her further life.

Mini transcript about finding values in the pain of loss

Therapist: During the treatment, you stood still and looked at different experiences from your past from a distance. What have you discovered in how others interacted with you?

Client: I never felt like I mattered. What I said or felt ... no one really paid attention to that. My parents were mainly concerned with taking care of my sister and working to earn enough money. The only way to get any attention was if I was good and did my best to help at home.

Therapist: What did you miss at that time that was important to you as a child?

Client: That my parents would have been there for me too. Would have interacted with me, not just when I was helping. Just that they also listened when I had something to say or comforted me when I felt sad or something.

Therapist: So, you missed the loving attention of your parents, who were mainly concerned with caring for your sick sister.

Client: Yes, very much so.

Therapist: What is that like to think about it?

Client: Painful. Sad. I would have loved for someone to have been there for me too.

Therapist: Someone who paid attention to your feelings and needs?

> *Client:*   Yes, that is not there now either. And yes, I don't draw any attention to it either. I'm always concerned with what it's like for others and whether I can do anything for them.
>
> *Therapist:*   Could we say that in your life now, it is important that people around you also pay attention to how you feel and what you need?
>
> *Client:*   Yes, that would be nice. I don't want to spend my life just being there for others and thus shortchanging myself.
>
> *Therapist:*   Could we see 'attention to your feelings and needs' as something valuable that you want to invest in your life for now and the future?
>
> *Client:*   Yes, absolutely. That is very important to me now.

If the client has missed something valuable or meaningful in his life or has lost it in some way, it affects him and hurts. That makes him sad; it makes him angry or anxious. Pain and values are therefore inextricably linked. In other words, in our pain, we find our values, and vice versa. As a therapist, you can therefore find an entry point to values by reflecting on the lack or loss of something valuable.

In direct contact with the experience of the painful and the valuable, the client also becomes motivated to pick up things that are valuable to him and shape them in some way. The client's past no longer determines his present and future. In his life story, he can find inspiration to see and feel what really matters to his life now and in the future.

Your client takes a look into the future

For many clients, it is difficult to know what they want to do differently in their lives. Rather, they are aiming at reducing their symptoms so that they can operate as usual. However, during treatment, they have discovered that how they have lived until now no longer works and certainly does not contribute to what they would like their life to be. So far, clients only know their story, and deviating from their known conclusions, beliefs, and rules feels uncomfortable. People tend to relapse into old, familiar habits.

A client who is usually reserved in social contacts will exceptionally respond openly and witty in the very familiar environment of his best friends. Yet he will generally show little of himself, rather listening to the stories and wishes of others and quickly apologizing if he expresses his own opinions bluntly. Clients often know very well what the boundaries are in which their story traps them. They lack insight into what they really want for their lives, now and in the future, because they no longer dare to think outside their storylines. The question of what is important to him can make the client feel as if he is lost and does not know how to proceed. The following metaphor can illustrate this feeling for your client.

Lost-in-the-mist metaphor

Losing what is valuable in our lives is like being lost on a boat at sea in a thick fog. The boat is at the mercy of the waves and currents. The fog is blinding, and it is then impossible to know where the land is and where the ocean is. Without a compass, the boat drifts around without direction. To know where we want to go again, we need a view of something that seems worth paddling to, even if it is foggy. Then, for example, the faint light of a lighthouse can provide direction, regardless of what obstacles remain along the way.

Values are like a lighthouse in the distance, from which you can determine your course. It is important that we gain insight into this.

We will have to create and clarify this perspective together with the client. To get an initial idea of who the client wants to be and where he wants to go with his life, it can be helpful to look into the future. In Chapter 7, the client learned to look at who he was in his past. Now he can see who he wants to be in the future. This offers a perspective that the client can focus on further.

We would like to invite you to do the following exercise for yourself and write down the answers to the questions.

Exercise

I want to look into the future with you. We have already looked extensively at and considered your experiences in your past. Who you were then and how you developed. Now let us look at who you want to be in the future. Imagine where you would like to be in five years. It can help to close your eyes for a moment and imagine your older self. You in five years. That may be the best possible version of yourself. How would you like to see yourself?
Look around you and consider a number of questions:

Who is with you?

....

....

....

....

Which people are important to you, and would you like to have close to you?

....

....

....

....

How do you want these people to see you?

....

....

....

....

How do you want to interact with these people?

....

....

....

....

In what way could you have grown further as a person?
    In your family, your work, your free time?

....

....

....

....

By focusing on these (or other) questions for a while, from the perspective of your 'older Self', you can experience that there is a future toward which you can focus your value-oriented actions. Important themes may arise that you can explore and deepen further.

    Take note of any conclusions and important themes that arise from answering the previous questions.

....

....

....

....

....

....

....

....

This view of the future offers you and your client, lost in the mist of his past, a bright spot on the horizon. The fog slowly clears, and many lighthouses become visible. They point in the direction of important areas of life that you can further explore together with the client.

Exploring valuable areas of life

For every person, there are many areas of life that are worth exploring. These areas of life can be relationships, parenting, family, friendships, work, leisure, community life, spirituality, culture, and nature. These areas constitute a wide landscape. Your values can act as a compass to determine which direction you want to move in these areas of life.

Exploring valuable areas of life can help your client to arrive at a broad and flexible behavioral repertoire. You can start with a general exploration of values and ask the client to reflect on what is valuable and meaningful in different areas of life. One way to start a conversation about this is to have the client bring photos (from booklets, from the internet, or homemade), quotes, or objects into the session to use these as a source of inspiration for further exploration of what values, qualities, visions, dreams, etc., are important to him. You invite him to bring something for each of his relevant life areas.

You can now also do this exercise. Choose an area of life and find a photo, quote, or object for it. Something that touches and inspires you. Take the time to reflect on what meanings this image or object evokes in you. The following questions can help you with this.

Exercise

Area of life:

....

....

Image, quote, or object:

....

....

What touches you about this image or object?

....

....

What does it remind you of?

....

....

What is it a symbol for?

....

....

What does it say about yourself?

....

....

What does it say about your relationships with significant others?

....

....

You can also do this reflection in other areas of life that are relevant to you. From this, you can distill values that have personal meaning for you (or your client). It sketches a spacious and colorful landscape, where the many values on the horizon can provide direction for exploring the question, 'Who do I want to be if...?'

Exploring the question 'Who do I want to be if...?'

As a therapist, I have always found this question very powerful, because in my opinion, it is a fundamental question that refers to something essential about yourself from which you, as a human being, can choose how to behave in relation to important others. It confronts myself as a therapist, and as a human being, with my own blind spots. Who am I in the eyes of others? Does that match how I see myself? And do I really want to be like that? Think about these questions yourself.

Exercise

Who am I in the eyes of my colleagues?

....

....

Does that match how I see myself?

....

....

Who do I want to be as a therapist for my colleagues?

....

....

Who am I in the eyes of the client?

....

....

Does that match how I see myself?

....

....

Who do I want to be as a therapist for my clients?

....

....

By regularly considering these questions, I offer myself the opportunity to consciously choose again and again: 'Who I want to be in relation to others'.

Your client now realizes that he no longer wants to keep repeating his old story and is looking for a version of himself where he can blossom (again) to become who he wants to be. Many problems that clients get stuck in are in the relational sphere. For example, they do not express their vulnerable feelings enough, causing relationships to remain superficial; they are stuck in feelings of guilt and shame about their past, which causes them to invest too little in contact with their partner and children; or they are overzealous and perfectionistic in their work, which brings them into conflict with colleagues and employer. This requires new behavior from your client, in which he will have to relate to significant others in a different way.

The client usually finds it difficult to know how he wants to be. It can be helpful to first consider how he has related to others so far in order to build a bridge to how he wants to relate to others from now on. The following dialogue is an example of how the question "Who do you want to be as a mother?" is considered.

Mini transcript about exploring 'Who do I want to be if...?'

Therapist: I would like to discuss with you how you want to further shape your life, now and in the future. As a guideline, we ask the question, 'Who do you want to be if...?' Let's look at an important role for you in your daily life. Which role do you want to look at first?

Client: My role as a mother is very important to me. I really want to deal with my children differently than I have done so far. I don't want to be so distant and harsh with them anymore. And certainly, I no longer explode so much when they don't do what I expect of them.

Therapist: This is clearly not the mother you want to be for your children. If you were to see through the eyes of your children, how would you want them to see you?

Client: Like a mother who is kind to them. Who plays with them and listens to them. Being there for them when they are having a hard time. And who can remain calm if they do something wrong.

Therapist: What would it be like for your children if they had a mother who treated them like this?

Client: They would feel more relaxed and happier. They would come to me more often when they feel sad. Then they would have a mother who is there for them; really sees and hears them.

Therapist: What would it mean to you if your children saw you like this? What if you related to them in this way?

Client: That would mean a lot to me. That's how I would like to be as a mother. Being able to really be there for them. Being able to really share things together.

Therapist: What would that mean for your relationship with your children?

Client: That we are there for each other. Really hearing and seeing each other. That feels like really being connected to each other. [Client is visibly affected]

Therapist: It touches you, doesn't it, when you say that.

Client: Yes...

Therapist: It feels to me like you want to be a very warm, involved, and loving mother.

Client: Yes, that's the mother I want to be!

Together with the client, you map out who she wants to be as a parent/partner/girlfriend/colleague, etc. This gives her insight into what she wants to choose in her relationship with significant others in her current life circumstances. It is a way in which the client defines herself in a new way: who am I in relation to others?

Your client begins to feel how important it is for her to become the person she really wants to be. On the one hand, this offers her motivation to do things differently, and on the other hand, it can give direction to her actions. This makes value work so powerful and necessary for sustainably changing the client's behavior.

To strengthen the impact of values on the (new) behavior of the client, it is important to fully experience what is valuable.

How can you strengthen the impact of values as a motivation for behavior?

What therapists sometimes struggle with when working with values is that they get stuck in the abstraction of formulated values. However, values are more than nice words. They should encourage (or motivate) the client to achieve sustainable behavioral change.

Values come to life when one experiences their personal meaning. In order for values to strengthen (or reinforce) behavior, the client must also consciously experience the effects of his behavior. It is like eating strawberry flavored ice cream. If you do that without paying attention and just swallow, you will not be able to taste what makes this strawberry ice cream so tasty for you. By really tasting and paying attention to what you taste, you will enjoy the experience of eating a strawberry ice cream, and you will be more likely to choose a strawberry ice cream next time. The same goes for values. Your client must 'taste' its meaning, that is, experience and live it.

We would like to invite you to 'taste' it yourself first. The following questions can help you get more in touch with the personally experienced meaning of your values. Make a note of what comes to mind when answering these questions. Take the time to fully feel what you experience.

Exercise: bringing your client more into the experience of values

1. What does [e.g., emotional connection] mean to you? Can you give an example of a time when you experienced this? Go back to that moment and see how you expressed it.

What was going through your mind? What did you experience (in your body)?

....

....

....

....

What was it like for the other person to notice that there was a greater emotional connection?

....

....

....

What did you notice with the other person?

....

....

....

....

2. Imagine that someone you love shares something vulnerable about themselves – something that touches you. What do you notice about yourself? What do you experience (in your body?)

....

....

....

....

How does it feel to be approached by the other person in this way?

....

....

....

....

What does it bring you in relation to the other person?

....

....

....

....

What is important and valuable about that?

....

....

....

....

3. What does it remind you of when you experience [e.g., emotional connection]. How does it make you feel?

....

....

....

....

4. Which image or song corresponds to what you experience when you feel [e.g., emotionally connected]?

....

....

....

....

These questions also reveal that values and committed actions are inextricably linked. Values provide possible directions for your client's behavior in which he wants to invest, in other words, values-oriented actions to which they want to commit.

In the next section, we emphasize how your client can exercise governance of his behavior, given the circumstances of his life here and now. How he can choose behavior that contributes to his (re)discovered life directions and how he can, through trial and error, commit himself to the newly chosen path.

Commitment to a values-oriented behavioral repertoire

ACT is essentially a form of behavioral therapy, and changing the client's behavior is central. It is therefore important for ACT therapists to translate values into a behavioral repertoire that serves the client's self-chosen life directions (values). This direct link between values and committed actions has always been essential for me as a behavioral therapist, at least in theory. However, putting theory into practice was not easy. How could I work with the client to move from abstractly formulated values to a concrete and flexible behavioral repertoire to which he would commit himself? I also encounter this challenge with fellow ACT therapists and supervisees. In the following paragraphs, I will show how we can link abstractly defined values to concrete behavioral change.

Now that your client has become more detached from his story, new possibilities become visible

The distinction that the client has learned to make between the perspective (self-as-context) on, and the content of his story (self-as-content) offers him a broader view of new possibilities to deal differently with challenging or problematic situations in his current living conditions. Once it is clear what the client values, the question immediately arises as to what behavior contributes to living according to his values.

What does 'living your values' require of you? Does it require you to adjust your current behavior? For example, working less time in the evenings so that you can also spend time with your family. Or does it require a completely new behavioral repertoire? For example, choosing a new hobby or sport. It may involve behavior that requires you to treat yourself differently, for example, taking time to relax and treating yourself to a healthy meal. Or to interact with others differently, for example, organizing a weekend away to surprise your partner.

Starting from your client's broad values exploration, you can work toward concrete values-oriented behavior. The following dialogue between client and therapist provides an example of how you can start translating abstract values into concrete actions.

Mini transcript about moving from abstract values to concrete actions

Therapist: Together we looked at which things are really important and valuable to you. Now I want to work with you to see how we can translate this into concrete behavior.

Client: That seems like a good idea, because I don't know how to do things differently.

Therapist: You indicated that you found the following values very important. Particularly within your family and also at work in contact with your colleagues: authentic connection, being seen, trust, openness, and honesty. Let's see what behavior you can connect to them.

Client:	I find that difficult. I want my children and husband to really see me so I can feel more connected.
Therapist:	That is indeed very important to you. How could the relationship with you and your family look different?
Client:	We could take more time to talk to each other.
Therapist:	And make that more specific. What could that look like?
Client:	I would like to stay at the table longer after dinner to hear how the day was for them.
Therapist:	And also, that they listen to your day?
Client:	Indeed!
Therapist:	So, spending more time each week with each other could be something that serves the values of being seen and connection.
Client:	Yes, indeed, I would like that, and it is really important for our family to do more.
Therapist:	Yes, and how much time would you like to spend on this? And do you want that every day?
Client:	Well, I understand that everyone still has an evening schedule, but I think it should be possible to spend an extra 15 minutes to half an hour at the table every weekday.
Therapist:	Possibly. That would be behavior that contributes to your values. What does it take to make this possible?
Client:	I think I should introduce that to the others.
Therapist:	That seems like a good first step. What would you like to say?
Client:	You mean that I also indicate why I think that is important?
Therapist:	I think it would be good to be open and honest about what your needs are, so that they can know that too.
Client:	Yes, that's true. I show myself more then, huh. And that also means being honest, yes.
Therapist:	With this behavior you serve several values at the same time: authentic connection, being seen, trust, openness, and honesty. And there may be more behaviors that can contribute to this. Let's explore this further.

In this example, a start has been made on concretizing value-oriented action. You can ask your client to notice if there are any moments between now and the next session where he exhibits behavior that feels value-oriented to him. In this way, he becomes more aware of the different behavioral options that contribute to his values-oriented life. You can expand this further together with your client. This is mainly about increasing variation in both values and behavioral options. Thus, many behaviors can serve many values. It is then possible that your client will see that important values in his life from his past and present can strengthen a broad behavioral repertoire. Especially if certain actions are no longer possible. For example, a client who can no longer play volleyball due to chronic pain. He can still serve the associated values – such as team spirit, friendship, growth, commitment, sportsmanship, and health – through different behavior. He can live these values by taking up other hobbies or sports or investing in his friendships in other ways. For example, by taking bike rides with an e-bike or taking cooking courses with a friend. It is up to the client to take steps in values-oriented action so that he can experience the consequences of his new behavior. Indeed, new behavior leads to different consequences.

Different behavior, different consequences

If we keep doing what we always do, we will keep getting what we always get. It is a bit simplistic, but it does indicate that if we really want to experience something different in our lives, it requires different behavior. For example, if the client learns to perform new behavior based on his values – authentic connection, being seen, trust, openness, and honesty – he will have to deviate from his old conclusion and rules. He will then start acting in a way that he is not used to. For example, he may take initiative in starting a conversation, go against someone else's request, or express vulnerable emotions. This new behavior has other consequences.

Others around him will not be used to this from him. Some may appreciate his candor and also share more of their own vulnerability. They can understand him, ask more about what he wants, and take that into account in the future. Still, others may respond with laughter and not take him seriously at first. If the client continues to choose for himself, regardless of the reactions of others, others can clearly see who he is, what he stands for, and what he needs. At the same time, he can learn that a rejection of his opinions and requests does not have to lead to a rejection of him as a person. People can disagree with each other. He puts himself more at the foreground, making himself visible and known. He lives his values, and regardless of the reaction of others, he stands up for himself.

In any case, his new behavior leads to new consequences for the relationship with oneself and others. And that is what makes the new behavior truly valuable.

How can the context help your client?

In ACT, people always talk about the interaction between behavior and context (behavior-in-context). Context can be anything. The culture and society in which you live, the physical environment (including your own body), the events of the moment, and the story of yourself with your entire life history – that gives meaning to how you perceive and experience your current circumstances.

All our behavior is therefore determined by the current context and by the story of our life history (the historical context) that colors the current circumstances. The client has, to a certain extent, 'liberated' himself from the influence of his story and has oriented himself toward new possibilities. He has found inspiration in his values and experiments with a (new) behavioral repertoire that provides him with new experiences. The context has therefore changed and immediately contributes to the change in his behavior. The change of behavior-in-context is gaining momentum. For example, a client who has sat passively at home for a long time with gloomy feelings and thoughts starts exercising again in a sports club. After a while, he notices that his body is in better condition, and he is gaining muscle strength. He has more energy and feels more vital. The context – his physical condition in this case – has changed and immediately has a positive influence on his further behavior. He will exercise more and take better care of himself. Symptoms of sadness decrease, and he becomes more eager to take up other social activities.

On the other hand, the client can also arrange his environment in such a way that it helps him to carry out his new behavior. For example, by making appointments with the sports club and putting them in his agenda. By making friends and exercising with others. By purchasing sports equipment and placing it in plain sight at home so that he is reminded to exercise at home and the resources for exercise are easily available. He can join certain sports groups on social media, where he can meet people who inspire and motivate him in his healthier lifestyle.

The most important context that is changed in an ACT treatment is that of self-as-context. From this place, anchored in the here and now, he can consciously notice his painful feelings and sabotaging thoughts (self-as-process), allow them instead of avoiding them (acceptance), distance from them (defusion), and choose to follow his value-oriented behavior, such as in the example of taking up sports and making friendly contacts. Commitment to value-oriented action will, in turn, also promote contact with self-as-context. The client is aware of his actions and their consequences. As therapists, we want to monitor and strengthen this ongoing process of consciously choosing and appreciating the consequences of his new behavior.

Since it is the context that provokes and reinforces your client's new behavior, it is important to include the context when experimenting with new behavior. Think extensively and investigate together with your client what the context looks like or what he can add or change to the context, so that it will help him perform the new behavior. In the following dialogue, you will see an example of how the therapist helps the client clarify the context.

Mini transcript on clarifying the context for new behavior

Therapist: You want to show yourself more. Take your own stage and no longer live your life behind the scenes.

Client: Yes, that is clear now. I've been there long enough, and it's only made me more lonely and unhappy.

Therapist:	And it was a safe place to be. Coming out from behind the scenes and onto the stage will be anxious for you.
Client:	[laughs] Yes, yes! But staying behind the scenes is really no longer an option.
Therapist:	Okay, so what is an option? Any idea what that could look like for you in your daily life? Taking your stage can be done in many ways, I think.
Client:	Um, indeed. I have an idea. When I go out with friends, I am the one who always listens to other people's stories, but I never broach a subject myself. I want to do that differently.
Therapist:	What do you mean? What would that look like?
Client:	This weekend we will go to the café together again. I then want to take the initiative to start a conversation.
Therapist:	And?
Client:	Um… isn't that enough?
Therapist:	It can help if it is as clear as possible what you are going to do and what the circumstances look like. What you think you will encounter and how you will deal with it.
Client:	Ah, okay. Well, we are going to our local café with our group of four on Saturday evening around eight o'clock. We always sit at the bar. I'm going to talk about a book I recently read. They know I like to read, but I never tell them anything about it.
Therapist:	Quite stressful, huh?
Client:	Yes, I can see myself wiggling on my stool. I always get a knot in my stomach. But yes, that may be the case, eh. And I'm not going to be guided by my lion tamer anymore.
Therapist:	I can totally see you doing it!

Your client learns to create a context in which his new behavior is more easily evoked, and he can also make a more conscious choice to perform this new behavior. In the next section, we will discuss another important element of the client's context, namely the people in his living environment.

Who do you need in your life now and in the future?

People can also help us continue on this new path. They are an essential part of our context. It takes courage to honestly consider how you want to relate to people who are important to you. How and in what way does the client want to relate to others? Would he like to open up more to significant others, or is he choosing to have less or no contact with someone who does not contribute to growth in his life?

One client can ask a friend to go to the sports club. Another client can have a conversation with his colleagues to clarify what he can or cannot do at work due to an illness. Or another client might consult with his partner about how he sees the upbringing of his children and what tasks both can take on. In some cases, it can also mean that he reconsiders certain relationships and reduces or even breaks off contact with certain people. A client who always has the feeling that he or she is only a listening ear for a friend's problems may decide to put the friendship on the back burner or even break off contact. He may choose to leave a relationship because he realizes that he is only staying with a partner because of an old rule of 'having to be available for someone else at all times' instead of choosing for himself out of a sense of loss of an emotional connection with this partner.

As a therapist, you can ask yourself similar questions. Who do you need in your professional relationships and work field? Think about the following questions and write down what comes up.

Exercise

How do I connect with and relate to colleagues?

....

....

....

....

Do I feel safe sharing vulnerabilities?

....

....

....

....

Do I have people around me who can help me be the best therapist possible?

....

....

....

....

Who do I need to help me grow as a therapist (and as a person)?

....

....

....

....

How do I behave toward colleagues?

....

....

....

....

How do I relate to others on social media?

....

....

....

....

As a therapist, it is also important to take good care of yourself. You can be your best version as a therapist if you have a context (including other people) that supports you and in which you feel you can grow further. The same goes for your client.

Trial and error

The client must exercise governance of his valuable life

If you explore possible values with your client early in treatment, you run the risk that your client will identify values that are not really self-chosen but are based on the expectations, rules, and norms of others or society. He lives by the values of others and has never or hardly learned to think about what he himself considers important or valuable. He has previously learned to ignore his own feelings and needs and to focus mainly on what others feel or think. He has not learned to choose based on what really matters to him. The therapist is then the latest person to whom he will tailor his behavior in thinking, speaking, and acting. In other words, he tends to do and say what he thinks the therapist expects or wants from him. At the beginning of the treatment, this can strengthen the relationship between therapist and client, and you can give more guidance on the direction of your ACT treatment. For example, in entering dialogue about his story, going along with exercises and explorations during the session, or doing the interventions offered outside the session. But ultimately, we want to return governance over actions and choice of actions to the client.

At the beginning of the treatment, the client has lost control of his life and feels hopeless in finding a movement or direction other than that dictated by his story. During the values exploration and connecting appropriate behavioral choices, we as therapists must maintain the clarity of mind to see that the values chosen by the client are really his. Regardless of whether these are prompted or shared by others. He may learn that his own choices and motivation for his behavior are his own and that he is in charge of his life.

Learning to choose a life based on yourself, where your 'own values' come first and you exercise governance and responsibility for your behavioral choices, is not an end point. On the contrary, this achievement is the beginning of looking at life in a different way and, like any skill, requires you to do this repeatedly. Every moment is a new moment where choices have to be made.

Choose again and again regardless of the obstacles your client encounters

When your client connects with the stable psychological place of his self-as-context, he, as the owner (librarian) of the content of his story, can learn to use his actions flexibly in the service of a life that is meaningful and valuable to him. However, this is easier said than done. Although recognizing his story and how it defines him ("How his head determines where he places his feet") is a necessary condition for changing his behavior, it is not sufficient. The client also needs to know what behavior he wants to maintain or change in an ongoing pursuit of what makes his life worth living. Moreover, and even more challenging, is actually changing his own behavior in a sustainable way for the long term. Your client may learn to continue to choose to do things that make him and his life valuable.

When acting value-oriented, he will inevitably be confronted with unwanted and sabotaging thoughts, feelings, and sensations. His actions are then again dictated by his book (story) instead of free choice from his position as librarian (self-as-context). This can feel to the client as if he is back at square one. For example, a client who fears judgment from others may be affected by critical comments from a partner in a painful part of his story. Painful thoughts and feelings arise, and he tends to avoid them by withdrawing and shutting down.

This is all too human and requires patience and a compassionate attitude from both the therapist and the client. Living and acting from your free self-as-context involves trial and error. Seeing with gentleness and recognizing that this happens and is part of it can bring the client back into contact with the many things he has already learned during the treatment. He can then more easily cross the bridge from content to context and choose again and again to invest in a life where he can 'become who he wants to be and be who he wants to become'.

Case Lisa: part 2

On the theme of values and committed actions, I first discussed with Lisa her painful feelings of loneliness and the lack of more intimate friendships. I explored what it had been like for her to have missed the warm connection with her parents. How she had experienced rare moments of attention and care with her grandmother, even when she felt sad or scared. Lisa was increasingly able to encounter the loss and, at the same time, her need for real connection, emotional contact, sharing feelings and needs, and being seen for who she is in her qualities and vulnerabilities, not only her intellect. At home, she started to pay attention to the moments when she experienced feelings of loneliness and loss and how this also brought her into contact with her needs and with the value of offering herself what she had missed.

Lisa had experienced that she no longer wanted to go through life as 'her younger version'. She was tired of her story that she had lived thus far. She reflected on her 'future Self' and saw herself as someone who was really in contact with others. This image inspired and motivated her to let go of her story and make a more conscious choice to connect with others in a different way. We explored the question of who she wants to be in relation to herself, her friends, and colleagues. She made a collage of photos and quotes that depicted important values for her. She wanted to be someone who could make real emotional connections. That she could share vulnerabilities, but also that she wanted to show more of herself. Not only did she feel it was important to be there for others, but she also felt the need for others to be there for her.

We explored what behavior was needed for these values to flourish. During the session, I took the time to let her talk more about issues that interested her and explicitly asked her to express her feelings and thoughts about them. At home, she met more often with friends and even with colleagues. She shared what was on her mind or what she felt about certain matters. Her new behavior clearly had other consequences as well. Her friends said that they really got to know her. They liked that she also dared to be vulnerable and not just be 'the smart girl'. She also took a cooking course, where she met new people.

Yet it remains challenging for Lisa to make herself visible every time. Her story, with her feelings of insecurity, the idea of being 'uninteresting and unimportant' surfaces every so often. She then starts worrying again about what others think of her and that they will still think she is weird.

It is as if she is waking up again and again in the larger perspective of self-as-context and sees that, as a librarian, she has the choice to choose to follow her book (story) or to choose behavior that, with every step, brings her more into contact with what makes her life meaningful and valuable to her. It is up to her to continue to choose where she wants her life to go.

Summary and conclusions

In this chapter, we have seen how you can help your client to investigate what makes his life worth living in relation to himself and others and how he can put his behavioral choices at the service of a life that is meaningful and valuable to him. By exploring his story (self-as-content), the client has gained more insight into what he no longer wants for his life. From being anchored in his overarching, all-encompassing I-here-now perspective (self-as-context), he can now make conscious and more free choices. He can explore the question, 'Who do I actually want to be?' for his life now and the future.

We first saw what we mean by values and how they are linked to committed action. Both are inextricably linked, and we have called it value-oriented action. We talked about committing to actions that contribute to what makes life meaningful and valuable for the client. Values are abstract concepts that motivate him to act in a self-chosen direction. They are not focused on achieving a specific goal or outcome. The why of the behavior and the behavior itself is what is valuable, regardless of the outcome of his actions. This makes values-oriented action resistant to the vagaries of life and the inevitable confrontation with painful thoughts and feelings, which will always be part of his story and learning history.

In the metaphor of 'your life as a librarian', the client is anchored in his self-as-context, the place from which he can investigate how he wants his life to continue, and which behavioral choices are worth investing in. We started this investigation with the client by reflecting on the pain of losing or missing out on something that is of value in his life. In this pain, he can directly experience what is essentially meaningful and valuable to him. This inspires and motivates your client to further explore how he wants to continue with his life now and in the future. The imagination exercise, such as 'looking at yourself in the future,' offers him a perspective on an image of the future that he would like to strive for. It opens the eyes to a perspective and a direction, out of the fog of being stuck in his story (metaphor 'lost in the fog'). Areas of life become visible on the horizon, with bright spots on which he can direct his actions. Photos, quotes, or objects can help the client put into words his inspirations, qualities, values, visions, and dreams.

Exploring values is crucial to motivating your client to try out new behavior and extend this to multiple areas of life that are relevant to him. To gain more insight into what this new behavior could look like, it is helpful to explore the question, 'Who do I actually want to be as a parent, partner, friend, daughter, colleague, etc.' in dialogue with your client? This provides therapist and client with the breeding ground to translate abstract values into concrete actions.

Building on this, we discussed how the client can build a new behavioral repertoire by discovering new possibilities with different consequences. His past no longer must determine his future, and he can make more conscious choices in his life, here and now. We have seen how you can help your client when he faces challenges to continually act consistently with his values, even if he is drawn back into his story. By clarifying and creating the context for his new behavior, he can strengthen the momentum of the change process of his behavior-in-context in a sustainable way. Your client learns to make more conscious contact with his current context and to consider who he needs to support his value-oriented actions.

We emphasize that it is the client who must exercise governance of his value-oriented behavioral choices. During the treatment, the therapist gradually hands over governance and responsibility to the client.

Finally, we have seen that your client must choose over and over again. On his new path in life, he inevitably encounters obstacles again, which bring him painful thoughts and feelings (content of his story). This is accompanied by a tendency to relapse into old behavior patterns (and story). In contact with his self-as-context, he, as the owner (librarian) of the content of his story, can, on the one hand, choose to act from his story or, on the other hand, to build a life where he – despite the inevitable and human trial and error – always exercises governance of his precious life again.

Chapter 9

Finally

Lieve Bruyninx

This is the book all of the authors wished we could have read at the beginning of our careers. Our goal with this book was to demonstrate that working connections between practice and science are possible without overloading the clinician with theory. We wanted to connect acceptance and commitment therapy (ACT) with its roots in behavioral therapy and relational frame theory in a way that remains practically and clinically relevant, and more importantly, that encourages the reader to keep looking for that connection in their own work.

By separating the self-as-content and self-as-context components, which are traditionally described as part of the same component, into two chapters, we wanted to emphasize the importance of 'the story'. Clients and therapists are guided to a greater or lesser extent by 'the story' they have developed about themselves through their experiences. It's important for both of them to develop a perspective on how their story plays on them and how it pushes them in a direction that doesn't necessarily align with their values.

The importance of the story, which forms a central and defining part of the context in which the client functions, is crucial to understanding why clients persist in problematic behavior. This insight is necessary for the therapist, to be able to apply interventions tailored to the client, and for clients, to nurture more kindness toward their own stuckness and clumsiness.

It is always a challenge to offer exercises in a training or in a book. To be able to learn exercises, it is necessary for those to be offered in a structured way. Too often, clinicians will simply give their clients a printout of such an exercise or a worksheet to complete, or rigidly adhere to the structure of the exercise in their clinical conversations. We fully understand that, in order to learn something new, guidance and structure are important. However, we would like to reiterate here that the exercises in the book are more like indications than rigid prescriptions, and we hope that you will gradually make your own versions of them in your dialogues with your clients.

It is our hope that by first experiencing for yourself the exercises in this book, you will have gotten to know yourself better and that you will have been able to get a taste of how similar interventions can land with clients. We think it is essential that care providers be able to put themselves in their clients' shoes, because on the

DOI: 10.4324/9781032699691-10

one hand they struggle with the same universal human problems, and because, on the other hand, it is important to have a deep and personal knowledge of what you are asking of your clients. Becoming better aware of what is not working in our behavior is difficult. Changing that behavior is even more difficult. And it takes time. Many therapies aim to provide insight. ACT is a behavioral therapy, and that means that insight alone is not enough. It is important that clients be given time to develop the new skills needed to base their actions on their new insights. Depending on the treatment setting, it is not always possible to complete this entire process together with each client. It is precisely at such crossroads that it is important to share with our clients that change is a slow process, that it involves trial and error, and that their path of growth might take longer than the therapy trajectory.

Finally, we would like to emphasize that the well-being of care providers is of utmost importance to us. We cannot repeat enough times how important it is that care providers receive adequate care themselves, from themselves, from their colleagues, from their employers, and from people around them. Experiential work with colleagues is an important element to gain insight into your own patterns and to learn to detach your behavior from the influence of your story. Like therapists and their clients, "ACT books authors" are people who can get stuck. That is why we have readily shared our own struggles in this book, in the belief that you can relate to our quest. We hope this will help you take a gentle look at your own development and that it will help you become a better therapist, both for your clients and for yourself.

If you want to learn more about process-oriented work with ACT, you will find process-oriented ACT training courses and experiential workshops on our websites. The work of Robyn Walser is also very much in line with what we do. Finally, feel free to contact us directly with specific questions!

Lieve Bruyninx (Factorpsy.nl/En)
Yvonne Barnes-Holmes (PerspectivesIreland.com)
Ciara McEnteggart (PerspectivesIreland.com)
Roy Thewissen (In-cont-ACT.com)
Marjolein Vleugel (ExpertisecentrumACT.nl)

Thank you for reading our book. We wish you a lot of fun putting it into practice!

Index